LEARNING TO MASTER
YOUR CHRONIC PAIN

Robert N. Jamison, PhD

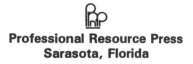

Professional Resource Press
Sarasota, Florida

Published by Professional Resource Press
(An imprint of Professional Resource Exchange, Inc.)
Post Office Box 15560
Sarasota, FL 34277-1560

To receive the latest Professional Resource Press catalog,
please call 1-800-443-3364, fax (941-343-9201),
write to the address above,
or visit our website (www.prpress.com).

This book was produced in the USA using a patented European binding tech-
nology called Otabind. We chose this unique binding because it allows pages
to lie flat for photocopying, is stronger than standard bindings for this purpose, and has numerous advantages over spiral-binding (e.g., less chance of
damage in shipping, no unsightly spiral marks on photocopies, and a spine
you can read when the book is on your bookshelf).

The copy editor for this book was David Anson, the managing editor was
Debbie Fink, the production coordinator was Laurie Girsch, and the cover
was created by Jami's Graphic Design.

Library of Congress Cataloging-in-Publication Data

Jamison, Robert N., date.
    Learning to master your chronic pain / Robert N. Jamison.
        p.   cm.
    ISBN 1-56887-019-1 (alk. paper)
        1. Chronic pain.   I. Title.
    RB127.J25 1996
    616'0472--dc20   96-15431
                                                      CIP

ISBN 13: 978-1-56887-019-9
ISBN 10: 1-56887-019-1

TABLE OF CONTENTS

APPENDICES *(Continued)*

PREFACE

Chronic pain is a complex phenomenon which can be influenced by personality, past experience, and present mood. One important component in gaining control over a persistent pain problem is to be as knowledgeable as possible about the condition and about the options for treatment. This book offers an opportunity for people with chronic pain to examine the various components of their pain problem and to gain a sense of mastery over this baffling phenomenon.

This book was written for use with a structured group-based pain management program. The topics have been selected to address those concerns of persons with chronic pain. Each topic can be discussed separately as part of a group session. Ideally, a therapist trained in pain management would facilitate the group sessions. However, this manual can also be used with pain support groups. The participants are encouraged to read the information before and after each session, complete the assignments, participate in the exercises and techniques, and use this as a reference guide should they experience a relapse in their condition.

This handbook has been created after years of experience in working with patients with persistent noncancer pain. The chapters were purposely written to be brief and easy to read. Each chapter can serve as an outline to accompany a detailed presentation by a therapist or group facilitator. The topics are suitable for presentation and discussion in a structured group-based program. At the beginning of each chapter is a brief overview of the important concepts to be covered. The topics in this manual do not follow a particular order, so a leader may choose to ignore some topics and spend more time on others. Also, the topics may not apply to all persons with chronic pain (i.e., persons with headaches may not have the same concerns as those with chronic low back pain). Group members are encouraged to review their own problem areas and to focus their attention on those topics which address these primary concerns. Professionals who interact with persons with chronic pain as part of their practice, such as general practitioners, anesthesiologists, neurologists, psychiatrists, psychologists, social workers, physical therapists, occupational therapists, and nurses, may find this book to be useful. A therapist's guide is also available to accompany this book with detailed strategies, suggested readings, and further information on organizing a structured, group-based pain program.

The field of pain management is not an exact science. As a result, there remain different biases about how pain should be managed. Often these biases reflect the field of training of the health professional giving the treatment. Attempts are made in this book to present the currently accepted pain management strategies with a behavioral medicine emphasis. One area of debate is how useful opioids are for treating chronic noncancer pain. Some practitioners strongly favor the use of opioids to increase the functioning of persons with chronic pain, while others feel that there is no role for opioids in noncancer chronic pain management. Until controlled studies can be done to determine the optimal treatment for persons with persistent noncancer pain, we can only encourage clinical caution and give guidelines as to how each treatment can be beneficial and/or problematic. Pain management is an ever-expanding area with new information being discovered all the time. It is important for those who deal with a chronic pain problem to be alert to this new information and to remain as informed as possible. Until the mystery of pain can be solved, we will look to management techniques in order to improve the quality of life of those individuals with persistent, unremitting pain.

The author would like to thank the many people who have directly and indirectly influenced this book, especially Gilbert Fanciullo, F. Michael Ferrante, Glenn Jamison, Wallace Jamison, Nathaniel Katz, Elizabeth Kay, Monica Micalles, Winston C. V. Parris, David Schwartz, and John Sullivan for their ideas and input. Thanks are extended to Julie McCoy, Jaylyn Olivo, and

Linda Gerry for their editorial and graphics help and to Giancarlo Del Vita for his imaginative cartoons. Also, special thanks to the faculty of the Department of Anesthesia, Brigham and Women's Hospital and the patients and staff of the Pain Management Center at Brigham and Women's Hospital, Boston, Massachusetts. This book is dedicated to the many patients who taught me much about living with chronic pain. Finally, appreciation is extended to my wife, Lisa, and our two children, Mary and Paul, for their emotional support and unwavering encouragement.

INTRODUCTION

If you have a pain problem that has lasted a long time and that is interfering with your life, this handbook should be helpful to you. It was written to be used as part of a structured program for persons with chronic pain difficulties like yours. The goals of the handbook are to help you to increase your ability to do things, improve your mood and your relations with other people, and educate you about how to reduce and control your pain. The best treatment approach involves a combination of exercise, group and individual counseling, and training in pain management.

Most likely you have been evaluated by a number of health specialists. It is possible that your doctor feels confident that enough healing has occurred to permit you to do more than you have previously been able to do. You have learned to protect parts of your body against pain and the risk of damage. Although it is difficult to learn to think and act differently, this handbook can show you how. You may be skeptical about the ability of these techniques to help you. You don't have to believe in them at the beginning for them to work. Whether they work and how well they work will depend on what you do after you begin, not on what you believe before you start.

At the center of any program are you and the other persons with chronic pain who may be with you. When you enter a program, you are setting out to bring about an important change in your life. The information in this manual and your participation in a pain program are likely to bring about that change successfully.

GOALS OF
MASTERING CHRONIC PAIN

These are some goals which a program may help you reach.

1. *Reduce Your Pain Intensity.* Patients have reported a reduction of their pain by 30% to 50%.
2. *Increase Your Physical Ability.* Patients have increased their physical strength and endurance by 50% to 100%.
3. *Control Your Use of Pain Medication.* After completing a program, patients have a better understanding of pain medication. Many patients either no longer use pain medication or use much less.
4. *Improve Your Sleep, Mood, and Relationships With Others.* Patients report that depression and problems in relating to other people are alleviated by 50% to 100%.
5. *Get You Back to Work.* Many patients whose goal is to return to work have been successful.

WILL A PAIN
PROGRAM WORK FOR ME?

This is a question often asked by individuals before they begin a pain management program. One way to respond to this question is to draw on past experience with patients who have attended pain programs. The following represents the top 10 ways to make sure that a pain program does *not* work for you:

1. Don't attend.
2. Try not to learn anything.
3. Don't do any of the exercises.
4. Don't try any of the techniques.
5. Keep a closed mind.
6. Resist change.
7. Look and act miserable.
8. Tell yourself "Nothing will help me."
9. Remain very serious and never smile.
10. Don't share anything.

A structured pain program *can* help you, but what is needed is your desire and willingness to try. With the help of your physician and pain therapist, you can get back in control and feel good about yourself again.

LEARNING TO MASTER YOUR CHRONIC PAIN

Chapter 1

PHYSIOLOGY OF PAIN

OVERVIEW

In this chapter you will learn about acute and chronic pain, medical assessment techniques, and the Gate Control Theory of pain.

ACUTE VERSUS CHRONIC PAIN

Acute pain is a sensation you feel when there is damage (or danger of damage) to your body. For example, placing your hand against a hot surface causes acute pain. The amount of acute pain you feel relates well to the amount of damage to the body. Acute pain gets better with time and medical care; it is expected eventually to go away completely. Resting an acute injury is important, and taking narcotic pain killers and tranquilizers may be appropriate.

Chronic pain goes on for months or years, continuing long after an acute injury should have healed. Chronic pain does not signal ongoing injury or damage, and the amount of pain you feel is not related to the amount of damage to the body. Chronic pain is a complicated disorder involving multiple systems of your body. Inactivity and pain killers help the pain only for a little while. Treatment of chronic pain involves close control of your medication and gradual increases in your level of physical activity. Initially you may feel worse rather than better when treatment for your chronic pain is begun.

The differences between acute pain and chronic pain can be summarized like this:

Acute Pain	**Chronic Pain**
New damage or injury	Old damage, no new injury
Improves with rest and time	Gets worse with rest and fluctuates over time
Activity interferes with recovery	Activity is necessary for recovery
Narcotics are needed	Control of medication is important
Short-term distress	Long-term stress and depression
Doctor "cures"	Patient and doctor work together

MEDICAL ASSESSMENT OF PAIN PROBLEMS

A primary interest of all patients with chronic pain is to pinpoint the cause. More often than not, no clear explanation for the pain can be determined. Many specialists rely on a comprehensive physical examination as well as different diagnostic tests. The following tests may be used to assess your pain condition:

1. *X-rays.* This test is useful in ruling out potentially life-threatening diseases such as cancer or tuberculosis. Plain film x-rays also allow the specialist to determine whether a degenerative condition exists in your bones which may account for your pain.

2. *Myelogram.* A myelogram is an x-ray technique specifically designed to determine problems in your back. A radiologist injects a dye in your spine to outline the spinal canal before taking an x-ray. Myelograms help to determine whether there is a narrowing of your spine or presence of a ruptured disc. Myelograms are being used less often because computerized axial tomography (CAT) scans and magnetic resonance imaging (MRI) are found to be superior tests.

3. *Computerized Axial Tomography (CAT) Scans.* CAT scans offer pictures of a "slice" of your body using computerized x-ray. Multiple images can be shown which allow the specialist to see different views of a painful area such as a back or a limb. This test is useful in determining structural damage due to a fracture, arthritis, a tumor, or an infection.

4. *Magnetic Resonance Imaging (MRI).* This test uses a computer and strong magnetic impulses to show images of your body. Results of MRI will allow you to see a large area of your body at once and help to determine problems with soft tissue such as muscles, tendons, and ligaments.

5. *Electromyogram (EMG).* This is a neurological test which uses needles and electrical impulses to measure nerve conduction. This is a useful test to determine gross nerve or muscle damage.

6. *Thermogram.* Thermograms are pictures of your body based on skin temperature. Areas which are cold are shown as one color while areas which are warm can be seen as another color. Thermograms are useful in determining problems with circulation and skin temperature changes associated with your pain.

These and other tests are most useful for ruling out problems which may account for your pain. They can offer peace of mind by telling you what you don't have. Unfortunately, many persons with chronic pain have normal test results. Also, abnormal findings cannot guarantee that a solution for the problem will be available. Because pain is a personal experience that cannot be accurately measured, the only "real" assessment of pain is what you say and what you do.

GATE CONTROL THEORY

Scientists view pain as subject to a kind of gate that can open and close, influencing which of the nerves' messages get to the brain for interpretation. The Gate Control Theory helps explain why, for example, you may not notice how much you are hurting during the day when you are distracted with other people but may be very aware of your pain when you are alone at night trying to get to sleep.

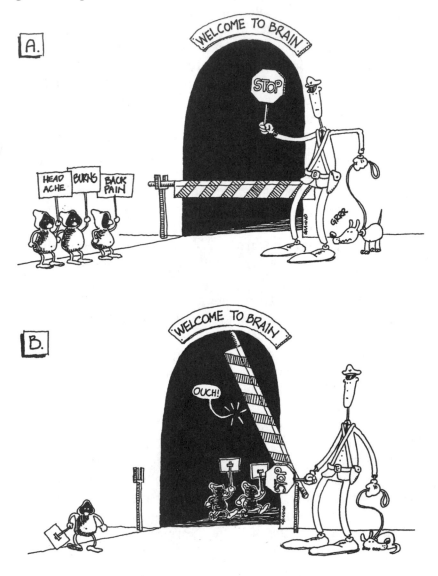

Messages travel with great speed from an injury to your brain. The messages are then interpreted by your brain, and you become aware of pain and discomfort. This pain warns you of danger and possible further damage. However, the messages coming to the brain from your muscles, skin, ligaments, and internal organs are only one ingredient in determining how much you suffer. The messages running up to your brain are, in fact, influenced by messages coming down from your brain.

FACTORS INFLUENCING PAIN

Pain is clearly affected by many factors other than the extent of an injury. Some of the factors that reduce pain (in other words that "close the gate") include the following:

1. Physical factors

   • Drugs (opioids, tranquilizers, anti-inflammatories, etc.)
   • Stimulation (heat, massage, acupuncture)
   • Surgery (e.g., cutting the nerve fiber or fusing the vertebrae)
   • Reduced muscle tension or arousal

2. Emotional factors

   • Relaxation and reduced anxiety
   • Increased optimism and pleasure
   • Social support
   • Emotional stability

3. Mental factors

   • Distractions
   • Humor and positive thinking
   • Active coping
   • Feelings of control

Complete the Daily Pain Rating Scale on page 201 while you participate in your pain management program. You should dis-

cover trends and changes over time which will help you in understanding and controlling your pain.

The most important points in this chapter that I want to remember are . . .

1. _____

_____

_____

_____

_____

_____

2. _____

_____

_____

_____

_____

_____

3. _____

_____

_____

_____

_____

_____

Chapter 2

RELAXATION TRAINING

OVERVIEW

This chapter presents different relaxation approaches to help in the management of your chronic pain. These specific approaches include (a) diaphragmatic breathing, (b) progressive muscle relaxation, (c) autogenic relaxation, (d) self-hypnosis, (e) biofeedback, and (f) cue-controlled relaxation.

DIAPHRAGMATIC BREATHING

Breathing is automatic - you breathe without thinking about it. However, you can train yourself to breathe in a way that helps you relax and reduces your pain. In fact, breathing is the basis for most relaxation techniques.

When you are in pain or under stress, your breathing often becomes quick and shallow. Unfortunately, this type of breathing gives you less oxygen, requires your chest and shoulder muscles to do more work, and can cause the muscles to tense up. In contrast, diaphragmatic breathing uses the muscles of the diaphragm and abdomen, not the chest.

Many people with chronic pain find this breathing technique to be helpful in learning to relax. Check your breathing every time you think about it. Watch what area rises the most when you take a deep breath - your chest or your stomach. With proper diaphragmatic breathing you should see your stomach come out when you inhale and go in when you exhale.

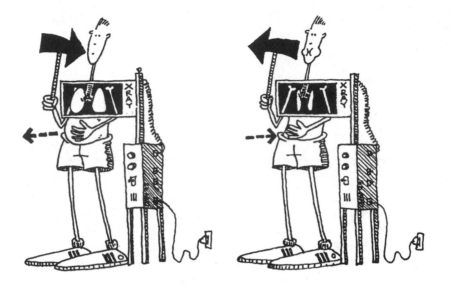

PROGRESSIVE
MUSCLE RELAXATION

Chronic pain tends to make your muscles chronically tense and tight. Progressive muscle relaxation is one way to learn to relax and control this muscle tension. Progressive muscle relaxation involves tensing and relaxing one group of muscles at a time. Do not tense your muscles to the point of pain or spasm. Only tense them enough to feel the tension. You should always be able to relax the muscles more completely afterwards.

Just like playing a musical instrument, relaxation is a skill. What is needed most is time and practice. Try to listen to a progressive muscle relaxation tape twice a day. It is fine to use this technique to help you fall asleep, but you should also practice at least once a day when you are awake and alert. As you gain skill, try relaxing muscle groups without the use of a relaxation tape. Periodically check those muscle groups which tend to stay most tense.

The following are muscle groups which are commonly tensed and relaxed to achieve a progressive relaxation state. First tense and relax each muscle group in the following order:

1. Make a fist with your right hand.
2. Tighten your right arm and biceps.
3. Make a fist with your left hand.
4. Tighten your left arm and biceps.
5. Wrinkle your forehead.
6. Squint your eyes and wrinkle your nose.
7. Tighten your mouth and clench your jaw.
8. Bend your head back.
9. Bend your head forward.
10. Shrug your shoulders.
11. Tighten your stomach muscles.
12. Tighten your hips and thighs.
13. Point your toes up towards your head.
14. Point your toes away from your head.
15. Curl your toes and lift your arches.

AUTOGENIC RELAXATION

Autogenic relaxation training is another relaxation technique emphasizing self-control. Unlike progressive muscle relaxation, autogenic relaxation is a passive technique in which you focus on certain parts of your body and imagine physical changes. You begin with slow, easy breathing and then repeat phrases in your mind that help you focus on sensations of heaviness and warmth, a slower heartbeat, and pleasant images.

The following are some phrases used in autogenic training. You may enjoy saying these phrases to yourself as part of your relaxation exercise program.

1. I feel quiet.
2. I am beginning to feel quite relaxed.
3. My right foot feels heavy and relaxed.
4. My left foot feels heavy and relaxed.
5. My knees and hips feel heavy, relaxed, and comfortable.
6. My stomach and chest feel heavy and relaxed.
7. My neck, jaw, and forehead feel completely relaxed.
8. They feel comfortable and smooth.
9. My right arm feels heavy and relaxed.
10. My left arm feels heavy and relaxed.

11. My right hand feels heavy and relaxed.
12. My left hand feels heavy and relaxed.
13. Both my hands feel heavy and relaxed.
14. My breathing is slow and deep.
15. My whole body is relaxed and comfortable.
16. My right arm is heavy and warm.
17. My left arm is heavy and warm.
18. My right hand is becoming warmer.
19. My left hand is becoming warmer.
20. Warmth is flowing into my hands; they are warm.
21. I can feel the warmth flowing down into my right hand.
22. I can feel the warmth flowing down into my left hand.
23. My heartbeat is calm and strong.
24. I am very quiet.
25. My hands are warm and heavy.
26. My breathing is slow and deep.
27. I am calm.

SELF-HYPNOSIS

Self-hypnosis is a way to help you to experience thoughts and images as if they were real. When you go to a movie you can allow yourself to be transformed into the lives and experiences of the persons that you see on the screen. By becoming mentally absorbed into the movie, you can leave yourself for a while and experience all of the emotions and activities of the actors. You can come back to yourself whenever you want, but you choose to experience other feelings and sensations. The same thing may happen when you are listening carefully to someone describe his or her experience of skating or playing ball. You can almost feel your body relive the experience of gliding on skates or hitting a ball while these actions are described.

A hypnotic experience does not mean that you are unconscious or asleep. People can experience self-hypnosis if they choose. Self-hypnosis is a skill that can be taught and may come easier for some than for others. Although some people are very "hypnotiz-able," others have difficulty experiencing hypnosis - just the way some people have artistic skills while others feel that they do not.

Some common misconceptions of hypnosis are that you will be put in a trance and that you will wake up not remembering what happened. Hypnosis does not make you do something that would be against your will. The most important part of self-hypnosis is that you are able to experience thoughts and images within yourself which make you feel better.

Self-hypnosis may consist of a series of suggestions such as arm lightness, deepening relaxation, and visualization of a pleasant scene. This must first be accomplished through listening to a hypnosis tape or learning a hypnosis procedure from a therapist. Unfortunately, self-hypnosis will not cure your pain or make it disappear, but it can allow you to "remove" yourself from your pain for an extended period.

An important part of the self-hypnosis procedure is concentration, lack of outside interference, and willingness to practice. There is a lot of evidence that self-hypnosis can be very useful in helping to manage a persistent pain problem. Discuss with your therapist whether self-hypnosis would be useful for you.

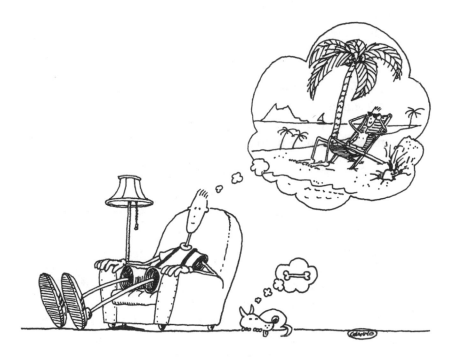

BIOFEEDBACK

Biofeedback is a treatment technique in which you are trained to improve your health by using signals from your own body. You have used biofeedback if you have ever taken your temperature or stepped on a scale. The thermometer tells you whether you are running a fever, a scale whether you have gained weight. Both devices "feed back" information about your body's condition. This information helps you take steps to improve your condition. When you are running a fever, you go to bed and drink plenty of fluids. When you gain weight, you go on a diet and resolve to eat less.

The biofeedback machine acts as a sixth sense that allows you to "see" or "hear" activity inside your body. Sensitive electronic instruments pick up various stress indicators in your body and give you information that helps you learn what makes your body tense and how you can relax it better. Like anyone learning a skill, you need to practice. By watching for changes on a plotted graph or listening for a change in a tone, you can make internal adjustments that alter the signal. Biofeedback does not do anything to you, but teaches you ways to help yourself. The biofeedback therapist acts as a coach, giving you tips on how to improve your performance.

Types of biofeedback include

1. *Electromyographic (EMG) Biofeedback.* EMG biofeedback measures muscle tension. Every time muscles contract, they give off a small electrical impulse. Tense muscles put out more electrical activity than relaxed muscles. In this type of biofeedback, electrodes that are placed on the skin sense the amount of electrical activity. As your muscles tighten up, this electrical activity increases; as they relax, it decreases. A biofeedback unit translates these signals into audible tones or visual displays that indicate the amount of muscle tension.

2. *Peripheral Temperature (TEMP).* This unit acts much like a thermometer. When you are tense or worried, the smooth muscles around your blood vessels constrict. This change contributes to coldness in your hands and your feet. Sensitive units that measure skin temperature indicate the amount of blood flow to your extremities. As

you tense up, the blood flow decreases and the temperature falls. As you relax, the blood flow increases and the temperature goes up.

3. *Electrodermal Activity (EDA)*. When you become tense and anxious, your sweat glands become more active. Sweaty skin conducts electricity better than dry skin. Thus, as you become tense, your skin conductance goes up; as you become more relaxed, your skin conductance goes down. An electrical unit measures electrodermal activity (the amount of perspiration given off in certain areas of the body), which serves as a measure of emotional excitability.

Other biofeedback units measure your heart rate, your breathing rate, or the electrical activity in your brain. All of these units give you information about what your body is doing. With this information, you learn to change and control some of the physical reactions that you have felt were uncontrollable.

People with chronic pain tend to brace or guard parts of their body and to remain on the alert because of their pain. Unfortunately, when you become tense or anxious, your pain tends to be worse. Biofeedback therapy gives you strategies to control the physiological reactions of your body, particularly when you're in pain. You may want to discuss with a biofeedback therapist whether you are a good candidate for biofeedback therapy.

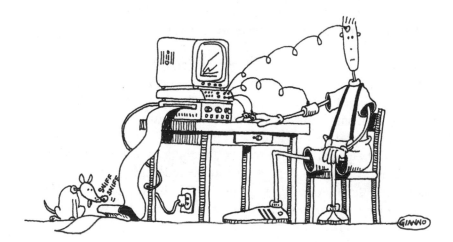

CUE-CONTROLLED RELAXATION

Once you have learned some relaxation techniques, through either progressive muscle relaxation or biofeedback, you will want to apply these relaxation skills in your everyday life. One technique is called cue-controlled relaxation. The steps to be taken in cue-controlled relaxation are

1. Recall what it felt like to release muscle tension during relaxation training and biofeedback therapy.
2. Begin to breathe in through your nose and out through your mouth. Gently blow most of the air out of your lungs; as you fill your lungs again, slightly push out your stomach, causing it to rise an inch or so. Try to avoid moving your chest or shoulders as you breathe in.
3. Continue to breathe in and out at a slow and regular rate. Breathe in for a count of 3, hold your breath for a moment, and breathe out for a count of about 6. While you are breathing out, your stomach should slowly go down.
4. As you focus on your breathing, begin to silently repeat the phrase "I am relaxed." Each time you breathe in, say to yourself "I am"; as you breath out, silently repeat "relaxed."

The key to effective cue-controlled relaxation is being able to pair the phrase "I am relaxed" with relaxed breathing exercises. Repeating this phrase and enjoying relaxed breathing can serve as "cues" in helping you to control your pain.

You can use cue-controlled relaxation as often as you like and just about anywhere. People use cue-controlled relaxation when they are driving, before or after doing something stressful, or off and on during the day. You may find that you don't feel quite as relaxed with cue-controlled relaxation as you might with a more involved relaxation exercise. Just the same, cue-controlled relaxation will help you achieve two of the goals of relaxation training. They are (a) to relax in a very short period, and (b) to be able to use your relaxation skills in your everyday life. The trick is to learn to be aware of your tension levels and to learn ways to relax periodically throughout the day.

The most important points in this chapter that I want to remember are . . .

1. _____

_____

_____

_____

_____

2. _____

_____

_____

_____

_____

3. _____

_____

_____

_____

_____

Chapter 3

EXERCISE AND PAIN

OVERVIEW

In this section you will learn about what it means to be fit, and you will review different types of exercises. Suggestions are given on how to begin a personal exercise program to combat your pain. Guidelines for stretching are included.

INTRODUCTION

Patients in pain are often instructed to rest and protect themselves even though the time when their injury should have healed has long since passed. In fact, prolonged bed rest can be detrimental in this situation because it is followed by a significant loss of protein and calcium from the body and a decrease in the productivity of the cardiovascular system. You need to move to keep the vital systems of your body functioning. Movement designed to increase your physical stamina is called "exercise." Exercise is also an excellent way to decrease anxiety, elevate mood, and control weight.

WHAT IS FITNESS?

Fitness is not necessarily having big muscles or looking tanned. There are five aspects to being fit:

1. *Cardiorespiratory Functioning* - the condition of your heart and lungs
2. *Muscle Strength* - the ability to exert a large amount of strength at one time
3. *Muscle Endurance* - the ability to contract your muscles to a moderate degree for an extended period
4. *Flexibility* - the amount of mobility in your joints and muscles
5. *Body Composition* - the amount of body fat (in women, usually between 16% and 35%; in men between 5% and 22%)

You need to consider all five aspects of fitness in order to be in good shape. If, for example, you are strong but you get out of breath easily, are overweight, and have tight muscles, you are not fit.

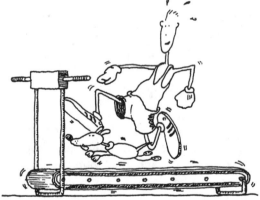

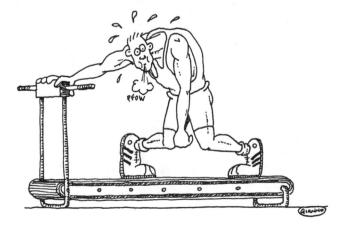

TYPES OF EXERCISES

Exercise falls into three categories:

1. *Type 1: Low Output Exercise.* This type of exercise includes stretching and gentle movement and is important in dealing with chronic pain. Regularly engaging in low-output exercise helps you improve or maintain your coordination, balance, agility, power, reaction time, and kinesthetic sense. Through this kind of activity, you also regain your confidence in your body's ability to move well.
2. *Type 2: Anaerobic Exercise.* "Anaerobic" means "without oxygen"; anaerobic exercise tends not to increase your breathing or heart rate appreciably. Anaerobic exercise requires movement over a short period (not more than 3 minutes). For example, you may need to climb a flight of steps or rush across a busy street.
3. *Type 3: Aerobic Exercise.* Aerobic exercise strengthens your respiratory muscles and the pumping efficiency of your heart. During aerobic exercise, your heart rate increases and you need more oxygen. Some of the best aerobic exercises are walking, cycling, rowing, and swimming.

YOUR PERSONAL
EXERCISE PROGRAM

In all three types of exercise, there are five areas of importance:

1. *Frequency.* You need to exercise frequently enough to benefit from the increased level of activity - perhaps three times each week.
2. *Intensity.* Intensity can be measured as how hard your heart works. Ideally, during exercise, your heart rate per minute is between 60% and 90% of your maximum desirable heart rate (which you can calculate by subtracting your age from 220).

3. *Duration.* Duration is how long you need to continue to exercise to benefit from the activity. Because movement tends to increase pain, it may be difficult for you to do any exercise for a prolonged period. Ideally, you will be able to work up to 20 minutes of activity at a time.

4. *Mode.* The mode is the type of activity you choose. You will need to experiment to find out which type of exercise works best without making your pain worse.

5. *Progression.* Progression means having a slow, steady plan for increasing your activity, including an initial stage of 1 to 4 weeks, an improvement stage of 1 to 6 months, and a maintenance stage.

Avoid disuse, misuse, or overuse of exercise. Setting realistic goals is important. A slow, systematic approach to exercise guarantees your safety while you work toward your goals. Here are some hints for your personal exercise program:

- *Get Started.* Find an exercise that you enjoy and can do on a regular basis. Schedule 20 to 30 minutes every other day just for stretching and exercise.

- *Start Slow.* Start at the level that is right for you. Gradually increase the duration and the intensity of your activity without overdoing it.

- *Don't Forget.* Link your exercise program with something that you do every day. For instance, do some exercises before you sit down for your special TV show. Everyday activities like walking your dog can become part of your exercise program.

- *Be Consistent.* If possible, do your exercise at the same time each day.

- *Record Your Progress.* Keep records of the type and duration of your exercise as well as how you feel both during and after each exercise session.

- *Vary Your Program.* Don't let boredom set in. Try different kinds of exercise. Exercise with a friend or a group of friends. Consider joining a health club in order to have access to a pool, exercise equipment, and aerobics classes.

• *Use Music*. Listening to music while you exercise can motivate you, stimulate you, keep your mind occupied, and provide an enjoyable rhythm.

Because you care about your body, you need to remain active to maintain strength and mobility. You also need to understand proper body mechanics and to use relaxation to pace your activities. Finally, you need to focus on your positive abilities rather than on your disabilities in order to improve your physical functioning and reduce your pain.

Complete the Daily Activity Record for 1 day and the Weekly Activity Record for 1 week found on pages 203 to 205. This will help you understand what your level of activity is now. Then use the Exercise Record on page 207 to monitor the progress of your exercise program.

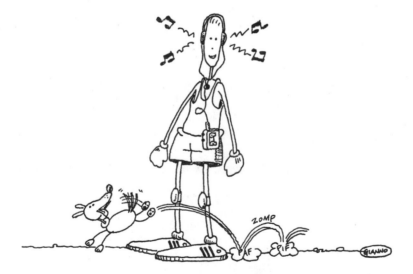

GENERAL STRETCHING GUIDELINES

Stretching is important if you are in chronic pain. The purposes of stretching are to increase and maintain flexibility and to prevent injury or cramping. You should stretch some every day. Here are some guidelines for stretching:

1. The correct way to stretch is

    •   Move into the stretch slowly.
    •   Hold the stretch for at least 10 seconds, then slowly
        release.
    •   Do not bounce.
    •   Keep your breathing slow, rhythmical, and controlled.

2. Holding the stretch for a longer period will increase your
    flexibility.   However, you should not hold a stretch for
    longer than 30 seconds.
3. Remember to stretch only until you feel a mild, comfort-
    able pull. Do not overstretch. Muscles respond to over-
    stretching by tightening up.
4. Wear relaxed, comfortable attire.
5. Be sure to stretch before and after exercise.
6. If maneuvering to perform a stretch causes pain, do not
    attempt the stretch.
7. If you have any questions or are not sure that you are
    performing a stretch correctly, speak with an exercise
    physiologist or physical therapist.

The stretches on pages 25 to 34 may be useful to you. It is important to first check with a physical therapist. He or she may not
recommend some of these stretches, instead substituting others.
Variations of these stretches may also be performed while you are
sitting or lying down.

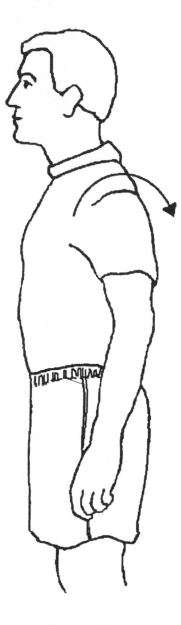

Stretch #1
SHOULDER ROLL

Standing as straight as you can, lift your shoulders straight up, back, and then down. Repeat 8 to 12 times. Do not let your shoulders come forward.

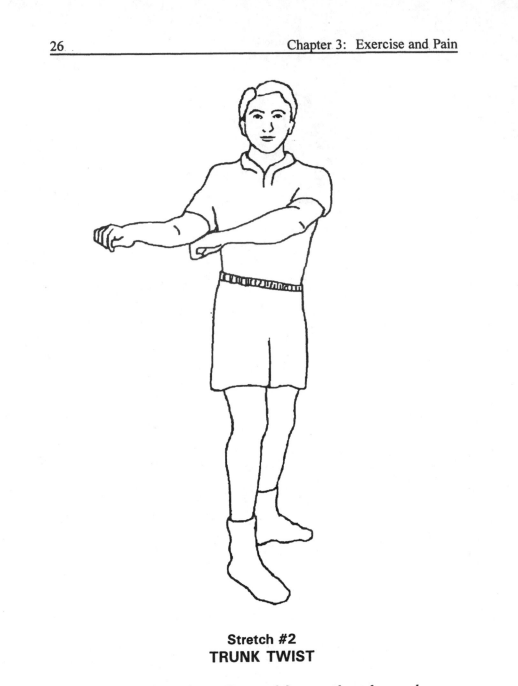

Stretch #2
TRUNK TWIST

*This stretch might not be good for you if you have a low
back pain problem. With your feet about shoulder width
apart and your arms extended slightly in front of you,
slowly turn to your right and hold for 1 second; then
rotate back to your left and hold for 1 second. Repeat
8 to 10 times.*

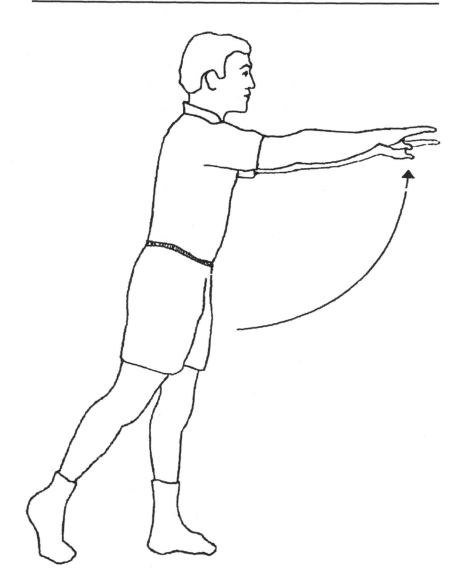

Stretch #3
CALF RAISE WITH ARM SWING

Stand with one leg back so that your heel is on the floor and your arms are by your side. Then lean forward as you swing your arms upward so that your heel comes off the floor. Lean back to the starting position. Repeat 8 to 10 times.

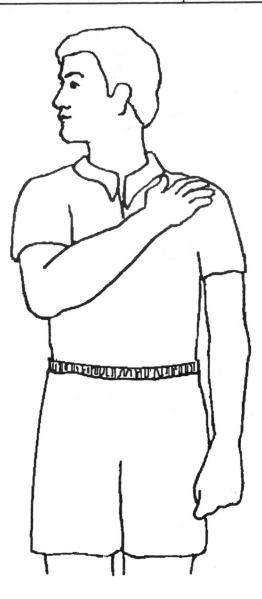

Stretch #4
NECK ROTATION

Placing one hand on your shoulder to prevent you from twisting, turn your head away from your hand. You should feel this stretch on the side of your neck opposite from the direction you are turning. Hold for 10 to 30 seconds and then switch sides.

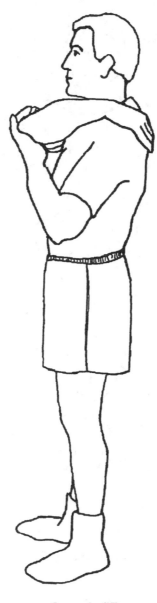

Stretch #5
FRONT ARM PULL

Standing as straight as you can, place one arm over your shoulder. With your other arm, push your elbow in towards your body. Hold for 10 to 30 seconds and repeat with your other arm.

A.

B.

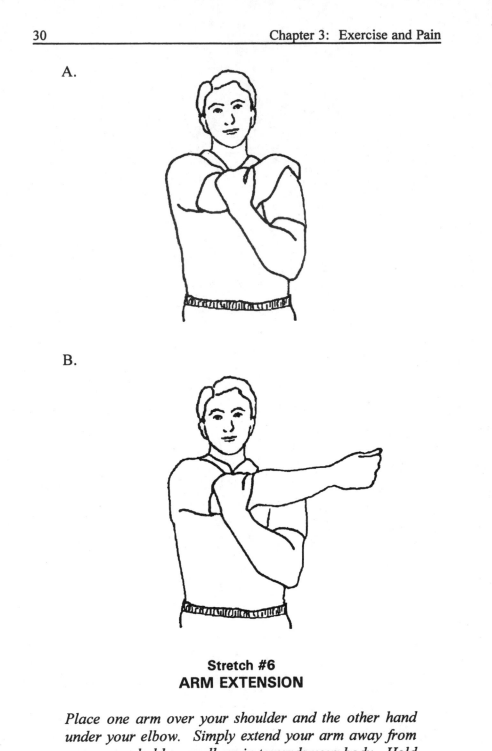

Stretch #6
ARM EXTENSION

Place one arm over your shoulder and the other hand under your elbow. Simply extend your arm away from you as you hold your elbow in towards your body. Hold for 10 to 30 seconds and then switch arms.

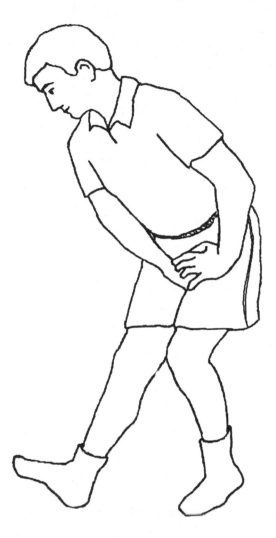

Stretch #7
HAMSTRING STRETCH

Extend one leg forward with your toes pointing upward. Bend your opposite leg and support your weight on that leg, placing both of your hands at the top of your thigh. Lean forward bending at your hips, not your waist. Keep your back in a straight line as best as you can while you bend forward. Hold the stretch for 10 to 30 seconds without bouncing. You should feel this stretch in the back of your extended leg.

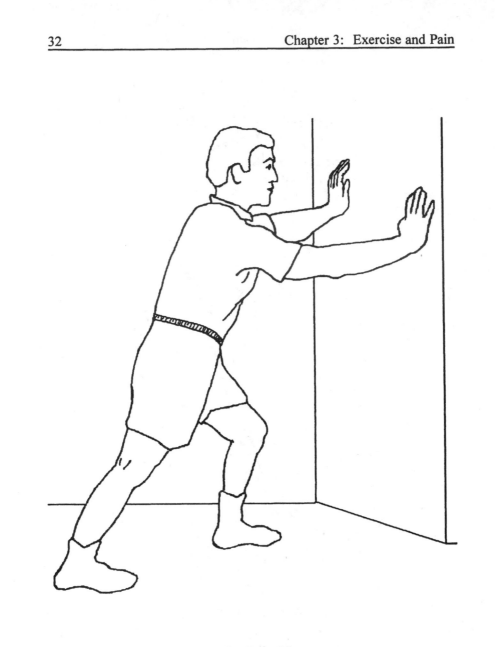

Stretch #8
CALF STRETCH

Facing the wall, extend one leg behind you as far as you can while keeping your heel on the floor. Lean forward into the wall and hold for 10 to 30 seconds. Just lean; don't push. You should feel this stretch in your upper calf.

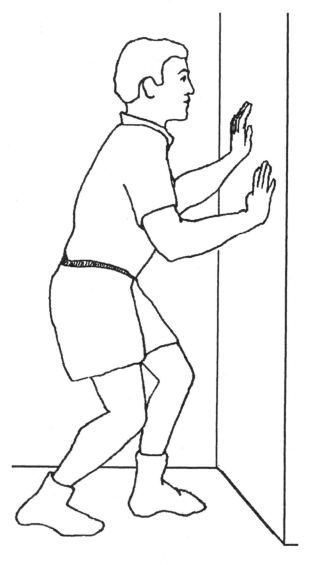

Stretch #9
LOWER CALF STRETCH

Face the wall with one foot 6 to 10 inches behind the other. Bend both of your knees and lean into the wall; don't push. Keep both heels on the floor. Hold this stretch for 10 to 30 seconds without bouncing. Switch the position of your feet and repeat. You should feel this stretch in the lower calf.

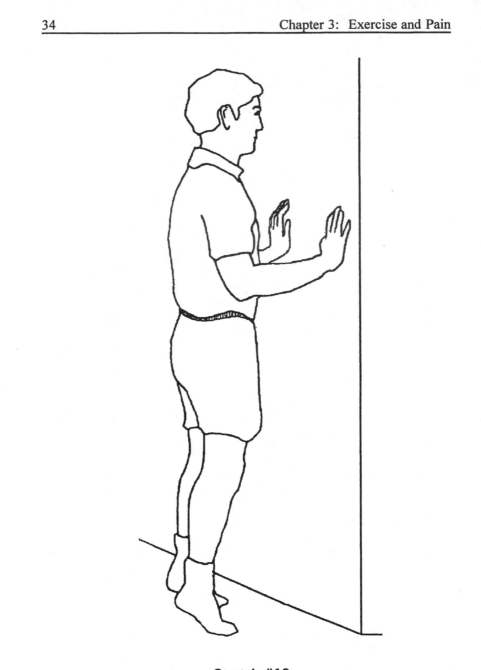

Stretch #10
CALF RAISE

Standing in front of a wall or behind a chair for balance, simply raise up on your toes and hold for 3 to 5 seconds. Repeat 8 to 10 times.

The most important points in this chapter that I want to remember are . . .

1. _____

_____

_____

_____

_____

2. _____

_____

_____

_____

_____

3. _____

_____

_____

_____

Chapter 4

POSTURE AND
BODY MECHANICS

OVERVIEW

This chapter explores how posture and clothing can influence your pain. Examples of correct and incorrect posture are given, and you can list factors which most influence your pain and how your pain interferes with your activities.

INTRODUCTION

Many pain specialists believe that pain can be either caused or made worse by bad posture, ill-chosen clothing, and poor body mechanics. "Posture" is the way you hold and position your body. "Body mechanics" refers to the way you move your body. In fact, patients with chronic pain frequently report problems due to activities that involve particular postures or movements, including sweeping the floor, vacuuming, getting in and out of cars, opening windows, doing dishes, emptying the dishwasher, or picking up laundry. Often these activities require bending and twisting, which are known to contribute to pain problems. In some cases, you may be able to change your posture in a way that enables you to engage in an activity without making your pain worse.

WHAT IS GOOD POSTURE?

The general rule of thumb for maintaining good posture is to keep your body as straight and "aligned" as possible. The following are some things to watch for in examining your posture and movement:

- Avoid bending forward or remaining in one position for long periods.
- Use arm and footrests whenever possible.
- Adjust your work surface so that you can maintain a comfortable, proper posture.
- Bend at the knees and keep your back as straight as possible when lifting and getting up.
- Avoid quick movements.
- Avoid twisting movements.
- Avoid overdoing any activity.
- Try sleeping on your side with knees bent.
- Be aware of the position of your neck as well as your back.
- Organize storage areas to prevent frequent bending or reaching.

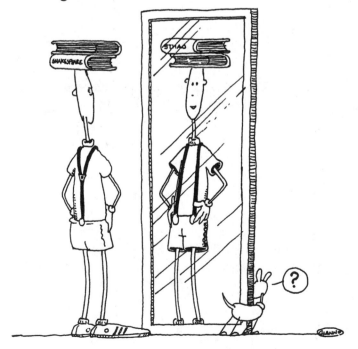

Examine the posture diagrams on pages 40-55 to understand the best postures to assume while standing, bending, lifting, sitting, and walking. Look at yourself in the mirror to see if you tend to lean to one side or to show signs of poor posture.

When you engage in any activity that can cause pain, remember to pace yourself: do a little bit at a time, and then rest for a short period. Also, don't be afraid to ask for help. If you know your limitations, you can often avoid short-term complications. The goal is for you to remain active and to maintain as normal a lifestyle as possible while avoiding or modifying those activities that contribute to your pain.

CLOTHING AND POSTURE

Clothes can make or break you in more ways than you may realize. In terms of your pain, what you put on your body may be as important as what you put into it. What is fashionable rarely coincides with what is comfortable to someone with chronic pain. What you wear and what you carry influence your posture and your movement. Over time, your clothing and accessories can have a substantial impact on your pain. Some of the more common culprits are tight jeans; belts that are too tight or worn in the wrong place; improperly fitting bras, pantyhose, tights, shoes, or socks; girdles; bulky wallets in hip pockets; and handbags and shoulder bags that weigh more than 2 pounds.

In addition, how you put on and take off clothing can affect your pain. Clothing that zips in the back, sweaters that pull over your head, and heavy overcoats require specific movements that may cause stress and strain.

Look in your closet and think through what you wear and how you get in and out of it. Tune in to how your body really feels in these clothes.

Complete the Clothing and Posture Worksheet (pp. 57-58) and the Activity List (pp. 59-60) to gain a better understanding of how posture and pain influence each other and affect what you can and cannot do. A worthwhile goal is to find ways to move as many activities as possible on the Activity List from the "cannot do" column to the "can always do" and "can sometimes do" columns.

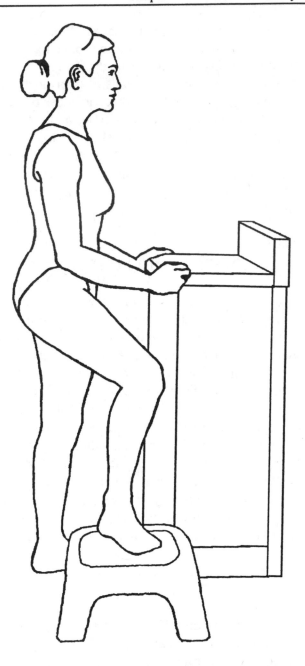

Posture #1
CORRECT POSTURE FOR STANDING

Use a footrest.

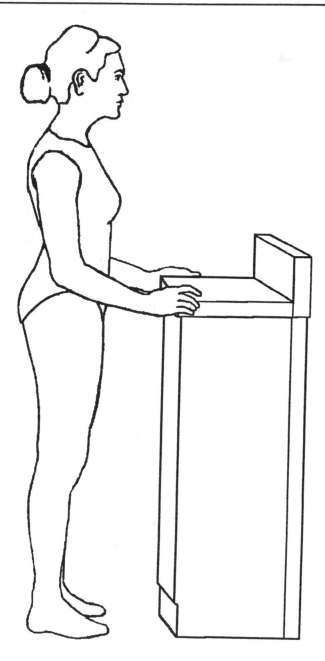

Posture #2
INCORRECT POSTURE FOR STANDING

If possible, try to elevate one leg.

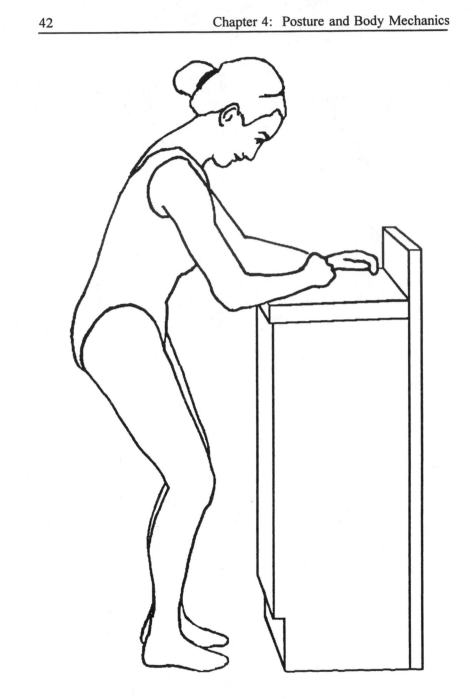

Posture #3
CORRECT LEANING

Keep your knees bent and your back straight.

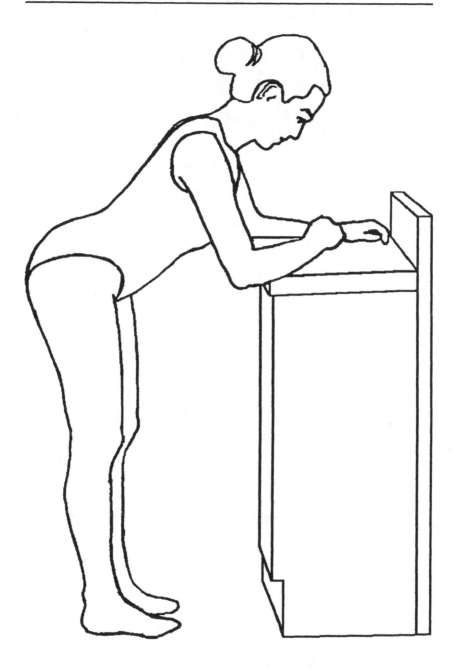

Posture #4
INCORRECT LEANING

Avoid keeping your legs straight and bending at the waist.

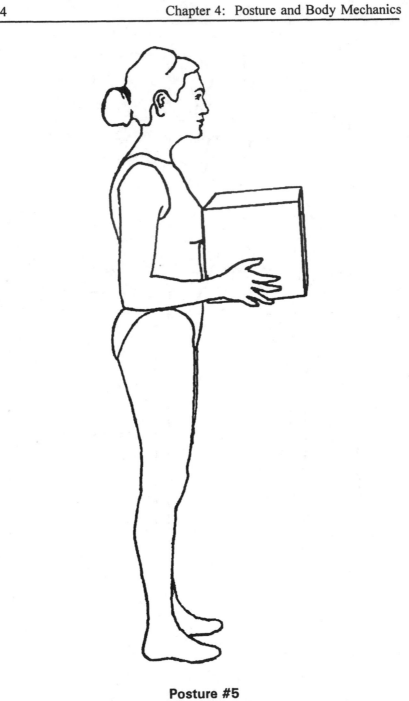

Posture #5
CORRECT HOLDING

Hold objects close to your body.

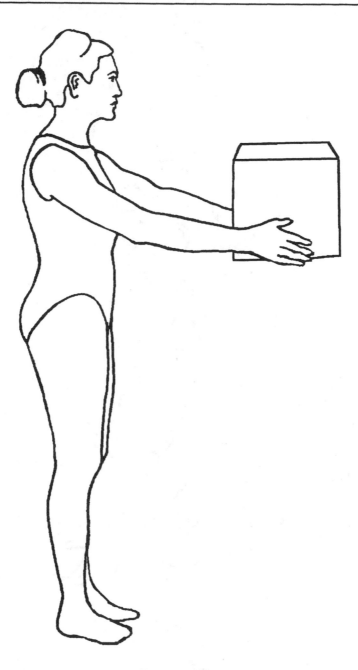

Posture #6
INCORRECT HOLDING

Do not carry objects with your arms extended.

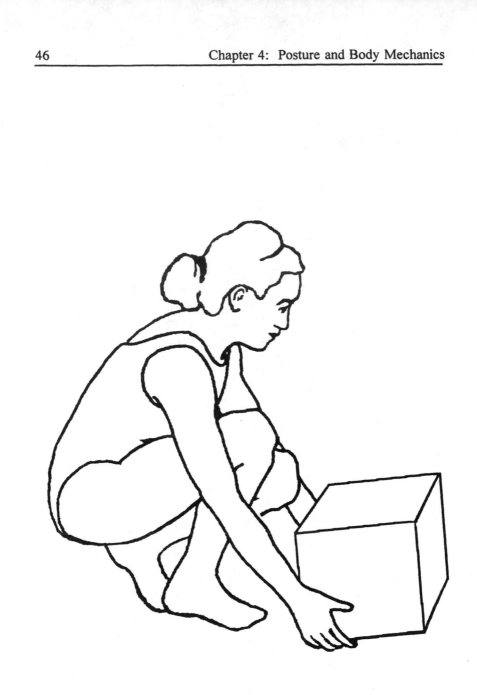

Posture #7
CORRECT LIFTING

Bend at the knees and lift keeping your back straight.

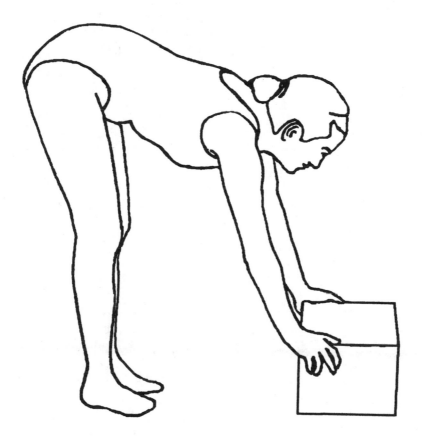

Posture #8
INCORRECT LIFTING

Avoid lifting with your back.

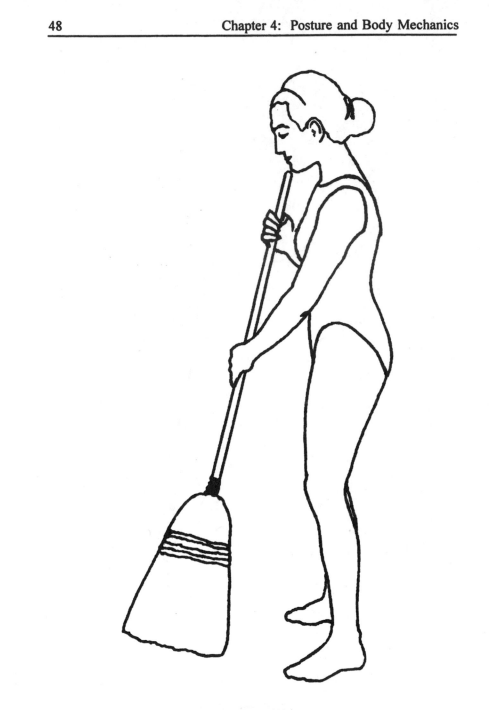

Posture #9
CORRECT POSTURE FOR SWEEPING

Keep your knees bent slightly and your back straight.

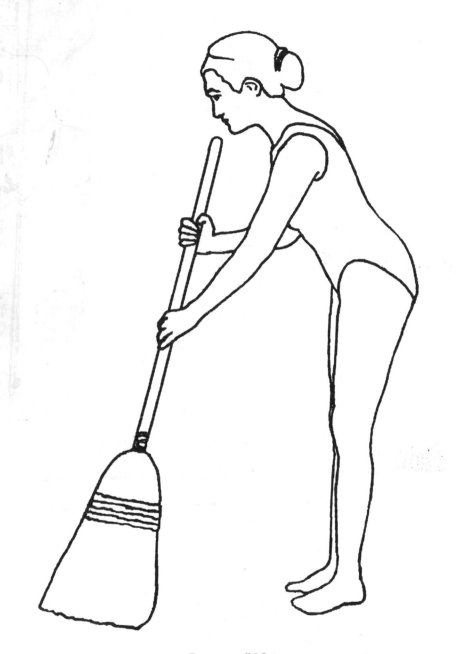

Posture #10
INCORRECT POSTURE FOR SWEEPING

Avoid bending at the waist.

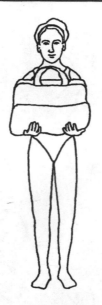

Posture #11
CORRECT HOLDING

Keep an object centered and balanced.

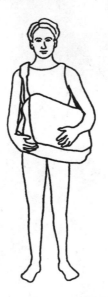

Posture #12
CORRECT HOLDING
WITH A SHOULDER STRAP

Use the strap across your body. Avoid using handles.

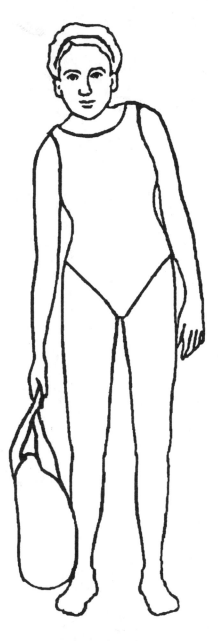

POSTURE #13
INCORRECT HOLDING

Avoid holding an object with one hand at the side of your body.

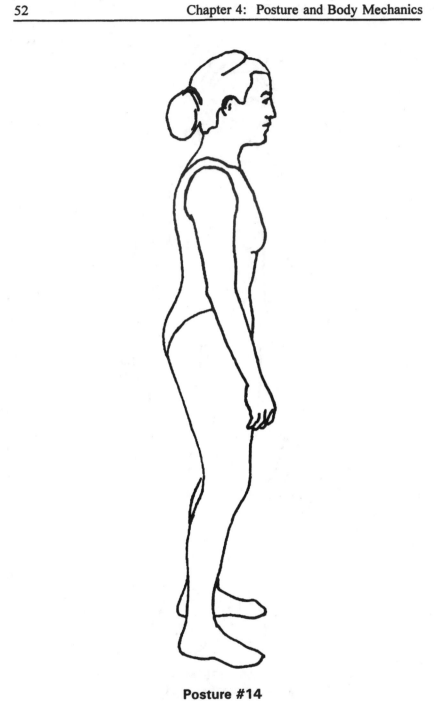

Posture #14
CORRECT POSTURE

Stand at ease with your back straight.

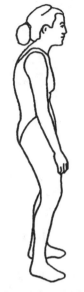

Posture #15
INCORRECT POSTURE

Avoid stooped shoulders with your head leaning forward.

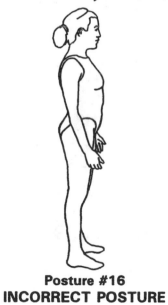

Posture #16
INCORRECT POSTURE

Avoid arching your lower back and holding a "military stance."

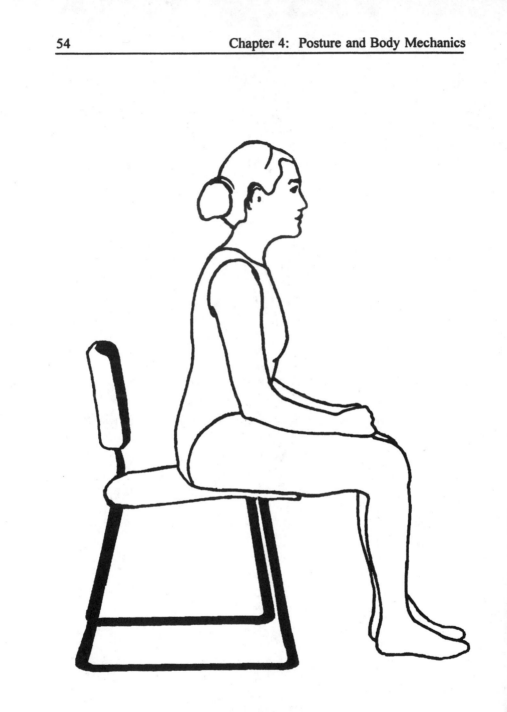

Posture #17
CORRECT SITTING

Keep your knees and hips level and your back straight.

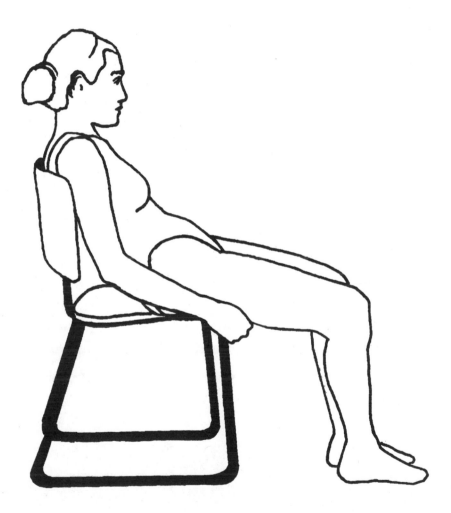

Posture #18
INCORRECT SITTING

Avoid slouching in the seat.

Clothing and Posture Worksheet

1. What clothing items and accessories make my pain worse?

    _____

    _____

    _____

    _____

2. What movements tend to make my pain worse?

    _____

    _____

    _____

    _____

3. How would I describe my posture?

    _____

    _____

    _____

    _____

    a. Do I tend to lean toward or favor one side?

        ❏ Yes   ❏ No

        Explain: _____

        _____

        _____

        _____

    b. Do some of my activities contribute to poor posture?

        ❏ Yes   ❏ No

        If yes, which ones? _____

        _____

        _____

        _____

c. Do some of my activities make my pain worse?

□ Yes   □ No

If yes, which ones? _____

_____

_____

_____

4. How do I usually lift, bend, walk, stand, sit, or get up from a chair?

_____

_____

_____

_____

5. What is my plan for maintaining good posture?

_____

_____

_____

_____

Activity List

On this page, make a list of specific activities that you were generally able to do in the past. These are grouped under work, household, outdoor, social, recreational, and sexual activities. Then, on the next page, place each activity into one of the following categories, depending on how your pain interferes with it now. Take some time to review this list. Over time see how many of these activities can be moved from the top of the page to the bottom.

ACTIVITIES I COULD DO IN THE PAST

Work
1._____
2._____
3._____

Household
1._____
2._____
3._____

Outdoor
1._____
2._____
3._____

Social
1._____
2._____
3._____

Recreational
1._____
2._____
3._____

Sexual
1._____
2._____
3._____

Other
1._____
2._____
3._____

MY ACTIVITIES NOW

_____
Date

Activities I cannot do:

1. _____
2. _____
3. _____
4. _____

Activities I should not do:

1. _____
2. _____
3. _____
4. _____

Activities I can sometimes do:

1. _____
2. _____
3. _____
4. _____

Activities I can always do:

1. _____
2. _____
3. _____
4. _____

The most important points in this chapter that I want to remember are . . .

1. _____

_____

_____

_____

_____

_____

2. _____

_____

_____

_____

_____

_____

3. _____

_____

_____

_____

_____

_____

Chapter 5

THE ROLE OF MEDICATION
IN CHRONIC PAIN

OVERVIEW

This section presents general information about medication for pain. Some common terms will be defined, and different classes of pain medication will be discussed.

PROBLEMS ASSOCIATED
WITH PAIN MEDICATION

Doctors hold many different opinions about the use of medication for chronic pain, and each doctor may give you a different prescription and different advice about its use. The reason for these differences is that the use of medication for chronic pain is very confusing. What may benefit you may not be helpful for someone else. Also, there are strong opinions of whether pain medication is good or bad for persons with chronic noncancer pain.

To help you sort things out, here are some terms doctors often use when discussing medication for pain:

1. *Tolerance.* Tolerance means that after you have taken a particular medication for a while, your body gets used to it,

63

and it becomes less effective. This may happen with opiod and tranquilizing medication. Surprisingly, some patients do not become tolerant to medications. Others, who become tolerant and who stop taking their prescription medication, report that their pain has not gotten worse and they have more benefit from over-the-counter medications.

2. *Physical Dependency.* You can become physically dependent on opiates, minor tranquilizers, and sleeping pills. In other words, your body comes to need a drug to function normally. Without the drug, your body goes into a state of withdrawal that is quite uncomfortable and sometimes dangerous. Most people can be safely withdrawn from a medication by gradually reducing the dose.

3. *Psychological Dependency.* Although physical dependency is traumatic, it can be treated and cured. A greater challenge is to overcome psychological dependency on drugs. This dependency may take the form of drug craving and thoughts such as "I can't live without my medication." Once you come to rely on medication, it is hard to manage without it.

4. *Addiction.* Being physically or psychologically dependent on medication does not mean that you are addicted. Addiction is often associated with legal problems which include getting prescriptions from many different physicians, forging prescriptions, and using medication for purposes other than pain control. Most people who take medication for their pain do not get into legal problems or show addictive behaviors.

5. *Adverse Effects.* Almost all medications have some side effects. The side effects associated with certain pain medications include drowsiness, nausea, constipation, unpleasant mood changes, dizziness, dry mouth, stomachaches, nightmares, sweating, difficulty urinating, weight gain, and problems with concentration and memory. These side effects eventually disappear as you stop taking the drugs.

6. *Illusion of Helping.* Medications for pain are not always helpful. Opioids and tranquilizers can deceive both the patient and the physician by creating an illusion of helping.

For example, some people will say that they drink alcohol to help them relax, to cheer them up, and to help them sleep. Most alcoholics will tell you, however, that they are often nervous, depressed, and unable to sleep. Similarly, in some people, opioids can increase pain, tranquilizers can cause anxiety, and sleeping pills can cause insomnia.

CLASSES OF PAIN MEDICATION

OPIOID ANALGESICS (PAIN KILLERS)

Drugs in the opiate family include codeine, Darvocet, Demerol, Dilaudid, methadone, MS Contin, Oramorph SR, Percocet, Talwin, Tylox, and Vicodin. The administration of opioids for chronic pain is restricted because of tolerance and dependency. In some cases, patients can manage well with regular opioids, while in others the need for the drug may add to the pain problem.

NONOPIOID ANALGESICS

For the majority of pain problems, aspirin, acetaminophen (Tylenol), and ibuprofen are useful analgesics. Nonsteroidal anti-inflammatory drugs (NSAIDS: Ansaid, Clinoril, Dolobid, Feldene, Motrin, and Naprosyn) help reduce pain and inflammation. Although in large doses these medications can lead to stomach problems and other side effects, they are generally safe if taken as directed. When these drugs are taken on a regular schedule rather than when pain demands, a small amount is usually needed and pain is more effectively relieved.

SEDATIVES AND HYPNOTIC DRUGS

These drugs (including Valium, Xanax, and other barbiturates) are given to help patients sleep, but this effect tends to wear off over time. If taken in increasing amounts, these agents can lead to dependency and addiction, and interfere with intellectual function.

ANTIDEPRESSANTS

The role of antidepressant medications in chronic pain is not fully understood; however, these medications (including Desyrel, Elavil, Pamelor, and Sinequan) can be highly beneficial to certain persons with chronic pain, often reestablishing a normal sleep pattern, producing an improved sense of well-being, and relieving pain. In low doses they are safe and do not lose their effectiveness.

OTHER MEDICATIONS

Other medications prescribed for persons with chronic pain include muscle relaxants, antipsychotic drugs, and antiepileptic medications. Unfortunately, some of these medications have limited benefit. If you have specific questions about medications, ask your physician or pharmacist. It is important for you to know what medications you are taking, what the side effects are, and how they will benefit you.

Record your hourly use of medication on the Daily Activity Record (pp. 203-204) and your weekly use of medication on the Medication Record (pp. 209-210). It will be useful to return to these records to track your progress.

The most important points in this chapter that I want to remember are . . .

1. _____

   _____

   _____

   _____

   _____

   _____

2. _____

   _____

   _____

   _____

   _____

   _____

3. _____

   _____

   _____

   _____

   _____

Chapter 6

STRESS AND
PAIN MANAGEMENT

OVERVIEW

In this chapter you will gain an understanding of what stress is. You will review some ways to break the pain/stress cycle, and you will be asked to complete a stress management checklist.

INTRODUCTION

Stress is the way you react physically and emotionally to change. Therefore, to deal with chronic pain, you need to know how much stress you can tolerate and how you can control your response to stress. Pain causes stress, and stress can increase pain.

Your physical stress response is automatic and can be positive or negative. Under normal stressful conditions your muscles tighten up, your heart rate and blood pressure increase, your breathing becomes shallow, your blood vessels become constricted, you perspire, and you often feel a gripping sensation in your stomach. This stress response prepares your body to meet an immediate, recognizable challenge. As soon as the challenge has been met or the threat has been dealt with, your body relaxes and returns to normal.

An abnormal or negative stress response is the same as the positive stress response except that you get stuck in the "on" position and cannot turn your response off. Smoking, relying on tranquilizers and muscle relaxants, and drinking alcohol do not relieve stress. In fact, these habits often add to the problem.

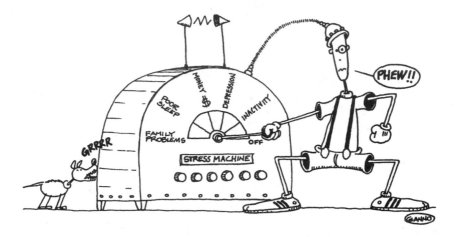

It is important to be able to "turn off" your stress response. Here are a few suggestions you can use to help break the cycle of negative stress and gain control of this reaction:

1. *Recognize Stress.* You may not realize how much stress you are under. Physical and emotional signals of a high level of stress may include increased irritability or depression, poor eating habits, fatigue, restlessness, and an inability to concentrate or remember things. The more readily you recognize these signs of stress in your body, the better you will be able to take action to alleviate your stress.

2. *Be Able to Predict Stress.* Anticipating problems can help you to handle them. Do what you can to limit stressful changes and to avoid hassles.

3. *Exercise Regularly.* Regular cardiovascular exercise helps loosen your muscles and decrease your level of emotional intensity. If you are in chronic pain, you probably hurt when you move, so you need to pace yourself and try not to do too much. Swimming, walking, and riding a stationary bike are all good forms of stress-reducing exercise.

4. *Change Your Environment.* Removing yourself temporarily from a difficult situation can reduce your level of stress and anxiety. Sometimes you may simply need to walk into the next room or say no to a commitment. At other times, you may need to make a major change in your life and environment. If you put some distance between yourself and a stressful situation, you may feel in greater control.

5. *Plan Your Day.* To feel in control of your life, you need to plan each day. Flare-ups in your pain can make your day unpredictable, so having a backup plan is important. Learn to pace yourself throughout the day so that you do not become overwhelmed. Take a break, sit down, relax, and then decide what you can manage today and what can wait until later.

6. *Get Some Support from Family or Friends.* Part of the stress brought on by pain has to do with the loneliness of the experience. Often friends and family members can be helpful. Learn to recognize when you need others around you for support or distraction and when you need to be alone.

7. *Learn Relaxation Techniques.* You cannot feel stressed and relaxed at the same time. By definition, relaxation counteracts stress. The many techniques used for relaxation include deep breathing, visualization, autogenic and progressive muscle relaxation, self-hypnosis, and sensate focusing. Relaxation tapes and soft, soothing music can help you to relax.

8. *Watch Your Diet.* Remember the old saying, "You are what you eat." Certain foods and eating habits can contribute to your pain and stress. Excessive weight gain can lead to poor self-esteem and greater pain. Avoid excessive use of salt, sugar, caffeine, and alcohol, and be sure that your diet includes enough proteins, dairy products, grains, and fresh fruits and vegetables. Specific information on proper dieting and nutrition for persons with chronic pain can be obtained from a pharmacist, a nutritionist, or your doctor. Your local library can also be an important source for information.

9. *Develop a Positive Attitude.* It is hard to be positive when you have chronic pain. Sometimes your mind can be your

own worst enemy. Recognize when you are in a cycle of negative or irrational thinking or jumping to the worst possible conclusions. Work to put yourself in a better frame of mind. It can help to share your thoughts with other people to get some perspective.

10. *Apply Problem-Solving Techniques.* You can reduce the stress you feel about future events by coming up with strategies you can use to cope with new difficulties. First identify the problem; then list possible solutions, think about each possibility, and try out the solutions that seem most promising. Problem-solving techniques help you to become somewhat "objective" about your problems and to feel more in control.

11. *Look for Gradual Improvement.* Like many people with chronic pain, you may feel impatient, hoping to find a quick and simple way to get yourself back to where you were before your pain began. Unfortunately, expecting miracles can lead to frustration and to an inability to come to terms with your pain. The best approach is to work for gradual improvements, recognizing that there will be ups and downs along the way.

12. *Be Aware of What You Cannot Control.* Because of your pain, you probably cannot do many things that you used to do. In trying to improve your situation, you need to recognize that some things are out of your control. Worrying about these things just makes your life harder. Periodically take a look at the things that are worrying you most, and figure out which of these things you can change and which you cannot.

13. *Seek Professional Assistance.* If all else fails and you feel that your stress is too much to cope with, get some help from professionals in the community or at your hospital. Sharing some of your concerns with a therapist or counselor can help you gain control of your situation and help you manage your chronic pain. Remember, you are not crazy, but your pain can make you feel as if you are going crazy. Getting some short-term help can make a big difference.

Complete the Stress Management Checklist on page 75. Think of a stressful event which may have recently happened to you.

Describe it and then answer the questions. Focus on those questions which were answered "no." How did this stressful event affect your pain? How could you have managed things differently? What will you do next time?

Stress Management Checklist

Think over the past few weeks, and recall a stressful event or a series of stressful events. Use this checklist to determine how you managed the event(s) at that time.

The stressful event(s) was(were)

_____

_____

_____

_____

_____

_____

_____

1.	Was I aware that I was stressed?	Yes	No
2.	Was I able to predict the stress?	Yes	No
3.	Was I able to avoid the stress?	Yes	No
4.	Was I able to control the pace of things?	Yes	No
5.	Did I have any outside support?	Yes	No
6.	Did I perceive things in a positive light?	Yes	No
7.	Did I deal with the stress directly?	Yes	No
8.	Were my expectations realistic?	Yes	No
9.	Did exercise help me manage the stress?	Yes	No
10.	Were relaxation strategies helpful?	Yes	No
11.	Did I eat well and avoid stimulants?	Yes	No
12.	Should I have sought more help?	Yes	No

Stress management strategies which would be most useful for me are . . .

1. _____

    _____

    _____

    _____

    _____

2. _____

    _____

    _____

    _____

    _____

3. _____

    _____

    _____

    _____

    _____

Chapter 7

SLEEP DISTURBANCES
AND PAIN

OVERVIEW

In this section you will understand the different stages of sleep and how lack of sleep can interfere with your coping with pain. Suggestions are given on how to get to sleep and how to stay asleep. Completing a Sleep Diary will help to identify particular sleep problem areas for you.

INTRODUCTION

If you have chronic insomnia (inability to sleep), you are in the company of 15 to 20 million other Americans. Persons with chronic pain often report that getting a good night's sleep is their number one problem. Although many people rely heavily on barbiturates, hypnotics, and alcohol to help them sleep, these drugs are seldom the answer to sleeping problems. Many of these drugs are highly habit-forming and must be taken in larger and larger doses to produce the same effect as time goes on. In addition, they can interfere with "deep sleep" or rapid-eye-movement (REM) sleep - a level of sleep in which you dream and your body gets recharged. Irritability, anxiety, and other psychological difficulties can result from these disruptions of normal sleep. It can be hard to stop taking these medications; you should do so only under medical supervision.

You go through four stages of sleep which can be measured by your brain-wave patterns. In stage 1, you feel drowsy, as if you are in a daydreaming state. In stage 2, you enter a light sleep from which you can be easily awakened. Stages 3 and 4 represent deep sleep in which you are unaware of what is happening around you. Unfortunately, chronic pain can prevent you from getting the deep sleep that you require. If so, you will feel tired and low in energy. People do not die from lack of sleep, and you can manage on limited amounts of sleep. However, improving your sleep will make a big difference in how you manage your pain.

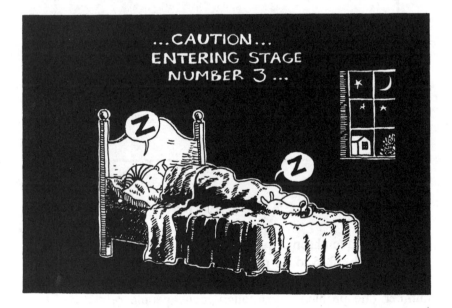

GETTING TO SLEEP

Although persons with chronic pain report having sleep disturbances throughout the night, getting to sleep is also a problem. Trying to fall asleep can be very counter-productive. The rule of thumb is to stop trying to fall asleep and instead create a condition in which sleep will occur naturally.

Here is one exercise to help you get to sleep: Set a pad of paper, a pencil, and a phone book on a table before you get ready to go to bed. Get into bed at your regular time. Give yourself 15 minutes to fall asleep. If you are still awake at the end of that time, get out of bed, go to the table, open the phone book to any page, and begin to copy the page just as it is printed. Continue to copy for 20 minutes. Then return to your bed and give yourself 15 minutes to fall asleep. Repeat the process if you have not fallen asleep in the allotted time, and continue to repeat it until you are finally able to get to sleep. Be sure to hold yourself to the time limit and to stick to it for as long as it takes. You will be surprised how helpful this procedure will be.

STRATEGIES TO IMPROVE SLEEP

If you are having problems sleeping, here are some suggestions that should help:

1. *Exercise.* Be as physically active as your condition allows you to be during the day. In this way you will have "earned" your sleep; in other words, your body will be tired enough for sleep.
2. *Relax Before Bed.* Allow a period of "winding down" for about 1 hour before bedtime. Do not engage in any strenuous activities during this hour. Ways to relax may include drinking something warm (not alcohol or caffeine), taking a warm bath, and using a relaxation tape. If you go to sleep and then wake up again in the middle of the night, you may want to repeat this procedure.
3. *Stick to a Schedule.* Schedule the same bedtime every night and get on a regular schedule. It is also wise to get up at the same time every morning. Even if you do not sleep well during the night, getting up at the usual time will make it much more likely that you will sleep well the following night.
4. *Stop Trying to Fall Asleep.* If you find yourself tossing and turning for more than 20 minutes, get up and do something relaxing until you feel sleepy again. Try to create conditions in which sleep will occur naturally.

5. *Avoid Naps.* Do not take unscheduled naps to make up for lost sleeping time. In fact, if you are having trouble sleeping, it is best to avoid taking daytime naps at all.

6. *Beds Are for Sleeping.* Use your bed only for sleeping and sexual activity. Reading, eating, and watching television in bed can condition your mind and body not to want to sleep there.

7. *Avoid Stimulants.* Avoid foods and drinks with caffeine for at least 4 hours before bed. Caffeine is found in coffee, tea, many cola drinks, and chocolate.

8. *Avoid Continual Use of Medication.* Don't rely heavily on tranquilizers and sleeping pills. When you stop taking drugs after using them for a period of time, it might take a long time for your sleep to return to normal.

If you follow all these instructions and still have persistent sleep problems, let your doctor or pain counselor know. You may benefit by keeping track of your sleep patterns. Complete the Sleep Diary (p. 83) for 1 week to figure out what may be contributing to your sleep disturbances.

Additional information is available for people who have persistent sleep problems. Consult your physician, pharmacist, psychologist, librarian, and people with chronic pain for more suggestions.

Sleep Diary

Directions: Please monitor your sleep behavior each day for 1 week. Complete each section in this diary.

DAYS	(Example) 1	1	2	3	4	5	6	7
DATE	10/20							
Avoided Day Naps (Y/N)	Y							
Exercised (Y/N)	Y							
Avoided Stimulants (Y/N)	Y							
Avoided Sleeping Medication (Y/N)	N							
Relaxed Before Bed (Y/N)	Y							
Used Distraction Techniques (Y/N)	Y							
Kept to a Schedule (Y/N)	Y							
Time to Bed (e.g., 11:00 p.m.)	10:00 p.m.							
Minutes to Get to Sleep	30							
Times Awake During the Night (0-4)	3							
Total Sleeping Time (Hours)	4 ½							
SLEEP SCORE (use scale below):	2							

(0 = Very Poor; 1 = Poor; 2 = Fair; 3 = Good; 4 = Excellent)

The most important points in this chapter that I want to remember are . . .

1. _____

   _____

   _____

   _____

   _____

2. _____

   _____

   _____

   _____

   _____

3. _____

   _____

   _____

   _____

   _____

Chapter 8

"COMFORT MEASURES" FOR PAIN

OVERVIEW

This chapter reviews a number of treatment strategies to help you through a particularly difficult pain episode. The strategies can be described as either "passive" (what can be done for you) or "active" (what you can do for yourself).

INTRODUCTION

At times, your pain may become particularly intense because of overexertion, emotional stress, the weather, or some other factor. On those occasions, you need a plan to get you through. Hopefully, you will have formed a "fallback plan" before the severe episodes occur. Keep in mind that the intensity of pain does vary and eventually will decrease. If possible, try the following comfort measures to prevent having to go to the hospital emergency room for an injection.

1. *Decreased Activity.* Limit your activity. Rest a little bit every hour. If necessary, use a timer to remind you to rest.
2. *Warmth.* Try using a heating pad, taking a warm bath or a hot shower, or applying athletic creams. Be careful not to burn yourself or to irritate your skin.

3. *Cold.* You may benefit from using cold packs and/or ice massage (in which you use frozen cups of ice with a popsicle stick to numb the area of pain). You may find it helpful to alternate between heat treatment and cold treatment.

4. *Electrical Stimulation.* Transcutaneous electrical nerve stimulators (TENS) placed around the painful area may provide some relief. If you have headaches, you may benefit from a pain suppressor which works like a TENS unit but is specifically designed for treating head pain.

5. *Magnetic Impulse.* Research is now being done on the use of high-powered magnets for pain relief. Quarter-sized magnets can be attached to the skin around the area of pain with surprising results. Units are also available which use magnetic impulse to treat headaches.

6. *Massage.* Try massaging the painful area while applying a warming cream. Use stretching techniques in combination with massage. Identifying trigger-point areas for massage can maximize the benefits.

7. *Stress Reduction:*

   • *Progressive Muscle Relaxation.* This technique, in which you practice tensing and relaxing muscle groups throughout the body, eventually allows you to relax quickly.

   • *Diaphragmatic Breathing.* Slowing down your breathing by using your diaphragm, gradually "inhaling relaxation" and "exhaling tension," sets the stage for generally relaxing all of your muscle groups.

   • *Imagery.* To help your mind relax, use your imagination to relive an event from the past or picture yourself somewhere comfortable and relaxing.

   • *Meditation.* Although meditation techniques are usually nonspecific, you can use them to focus your mind and to mentally remove your attention from the painful area.

   • *Self-Hypnosis.* Hypnosis incorporates the use of relaxation as well as self-statements, which have been shown to be useful in the management of pain. These techniques require some initial instruction and lots of practice.

- *Biofeedback.* In biofeedback, sensitive equipment is used to measure muscle tension, hand temperature, or skin conductance. The "feedback" you get from the equipment helps you to learn how to relax. After completing biofeedback training, you can relax without the equipment.
- *Sensate Focusing.* You can be trained to focus on an area of the body other than the painful site. This strategy, like other techniques of stress reduction, requires an amount of concentration that can be difficult to maintain when the pain is very intense.

8. *Acupressure.* You can get significant pain relief by applying pressure to certain points throughout the body. Specific "pressure points" are known to be related to pain in certain areas.

9. *Diet.* What you eat contributes to the intensity of your pain. Limiting the amount of caffeine you consume in coffee, soft drinks, and chocolate can help you be less anxious. Hot, spicy, and fatty foods may also increase pain intensity. Although people tend to smoke more when they are in pain, excessive smoking may also make pain worse.

10. *Distraction.* When your pain is intense, try to avoid focusing on it by getting involved in some activity, such as doing chores, going shopping, working on a puzzle, knitting, listening to your favorite music, reading, or watching television.

11. *Medication.* If necessary, opioid medication can help you through a particularly painful episode. Increasing doses of opioids may not be the answer for the long duration, but opiates can help when all else fails. You should first try nonopioid medications and share with your doctor what other strategies you have tried.

12. *Seek Support.* Intense pain can be a demoralizing, lonely experience. It often helps to share some of your feelings with other people and get some support. Consider forming a "support team" of people with chronic pain who can help each other at times when the pain is particularly intense and persistent. You may wish to contact a local

pain support group or call a national organization such as the American Chronic Pain Association (P.O. Box 850, Rocklin, CA 95677, [916] 632-0922), the American Pain Society (4700 W. Lake Avenue, Glenview, IL 60025-1489, [847] 375-4715), the International Pain Foundation (909 NE 43rd Street, Room 306, Seattle, WA 98105-6020, [206] 547-6409), or the National Chronic Pain Outreach Association, Inc. (7979 Old Georgetown Road, Suite 100, Bethesda, MD 20814, [301] 652-4948).

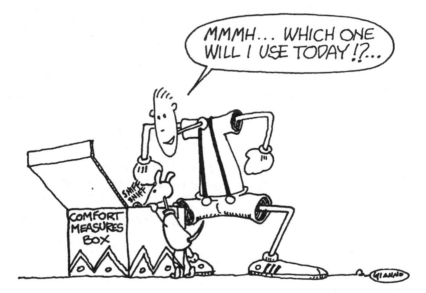

The most important points in this chapter that I want to remember are . . .

1. _____

   _____

   _____

   _____

   _____

2. _____

   _____

   _____

   _____

   _____

3. _____

   _____

   _____

   _____

   _____

Chapter 9

ASSERTIVENESS TRAINING

OVERVIEW

This chapter looks at communication styles and gives examples of aggressive, passive, and assertive responses. Suggestions are given in how to change the way you communicate to others about your pain.

INTRODUCTION

As a person with chronic pain, you may not be able to do everything that you used to do. Unfortunately, other people may not recognize your limitations and may tend to forget that you cannot do everything they can. Both of your two most obvious choices - constantly reminding people of your pain or doing whatever needs to be done despite your pain and eventually feeling resentful about it - are far from ideal. To handle this situation, you may need to change the way you communicate.

STYLES OF COMMUNICATION

There are three main styles of communication:

1. *Aggressive.* You act hostile. Examples of aggressive behavior are fighting, accusing, threatening, and generally stepping on others without regard for their feelings.

2. *Passive.* You hold back your thoughts and feelings. Ex-
    amples of passive behavior are not standing up for yourself,
    doing what you are told regardless of how you feel about
    it, and letting others decide everything for you.
3. *Assertive.* You stand up for yourself, expressing your true
    feelings in a positive manner. You act in your own interest
    and do not feel guilty about it.

Clearly, assertive communication is the most effective way to
get your point across. Assertiveness training has been found to be
helpful in dealing with depression, anger, resentment, and interpersonal anxiety, especially when these feelings have been brought
about by unfair circumstances. As a person with chronic pain,
you are the one who best understands your discomfort and your
needs. To help yourself, you need to be able to communicate
your feelings without passively collapsing or "blowing up."

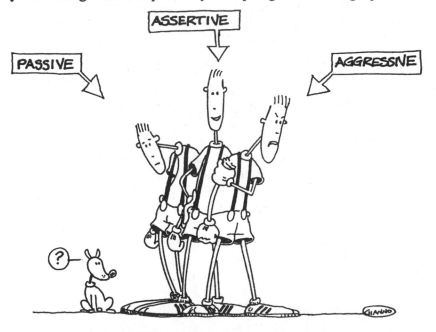

COMMUNICATING ASSERTIVELY:
TWO SAMPLE SCENARIOS

SCENARIO #1

You need to ask some of your fellow workers to do some
lifting for you because your back is hurting today.

Aggressive Style. "You never do much work around here. You know that my back hurts, and still you make me do all the lifting. People like you are the main reason that I have to suffer so much. So you better do the work, because I can't do it." (You are demanding, and don't care what others think or feel.)

Passive Style. "Do you think maybe, if it's okay, you could help lift something for me? I wouldn't have asked but if it's not a bother, I could use some help just this once, even though I guess I could do it, although I don't know if it's best for my back. So, perhaps. . . ." (You are afraid and worried about bothering anyone.)

Assertive Style. "We agreed that you could help me do some lifting on those days when my back pain is worse. I am worried about doing any lifting today. Could we trade jobs so that I can avoid having more problems with my back?" (You are definite and straight-forward. You make your feelings clear while making the other person feel listened to and respected.)

SCENARIO #2

You know that specific manipulations of your back and legs by your physical therapist are contributing to excruciating pain lasting for days after each session. Although you recognize the importance of stretching and exercising, you are not sure whether these manipulations are helping your condition. You don't know whether the therapist is aware of how much pain you are experiencing after your sessions. You are worried about discussing this problem with the therapist, but you decide that you will do so at the start of your next session.

Aggressive Style. "I can't stand your working on me any more. For days after these sessions I am barely able to move, and it's all because of your exercises. I want another physical therapist who will at least understand what agony I am being put through."

Passive Style. "I was wondering if maybe we could do less of the manipulation than we do, because I think that it may be causing me some more pain. Of course, you know best, but I was just wondering if these manipulations could be making me worse. What do you think?"

Assertive Style. "I know that you are trying to get me to increase my range of motion and improve my muscle tone. I also know that the exercises that you have me do are aggravating my condition. I would like to do the stretching by myself with your supervision. I will demonstrate my exercises and keep records if you watch and measure my improvement by the end of our sessions."

(Assertive communication helps solve the problem at hand. It makes you feel good about expressing your needs and encourages other people to feel involved and understood.)

IMPROVING YOUR ABILITY TO COMMUNICATE ABOUT YOUR PAIN

Here are some pointers on communicating with other people about your pain:

1. *Be Aware of Your Rights and Needs.* You, better than anyone else, know how your pain interferes with your activities. Be sure to separate your feelings and frustrations from your legitimate needs.

2. *Define the Problem.* In your own mind, define the problem and identify the factors associated with that problem. Be specific. Figure out who is involved in the situation and what makes it a problem for you.

3. *Decide on the Best Time and Place to Discuss the Problem.* Not all times are opportune for the discussion of an important topic. Ideally, you will have the other person's undivided attention and will be in a place where you won't be bothered by major distractions. Consider whether the other person's mood will promote a constructive discussion.

4. *Make Your Request.* Be as objective and rational as you can. State the problem and what you think would be a good solution. Be clear about what you would like the other person to do.

5. *Clarify Your Feelings.* Use specific "I" statements rather than talking in generalities or blaming others. Make your feelings known in a clear manner without being overly emotional.

6. *Follow Up the Discussion.* After a request has been made and/or an agreement has been reached, remind that person to be sure that your request has been heard or that changes are being made. Thank people who are helpful to you as a result of the discussion. Offer to return favors to express your appreciation.

Making changes in the way you interact with other people can be difficult. We get accustomed to certain ways of behaving and reacting. Because your pain may not allow you to do everything that you have done in the past, however, some changes may be necessary. Assertiveness training can help you feel good about yourself while minimizing problems with other people.

The most important points in this chapter that I want to remember are . . .

1. _____

_____

_____

_____

_____

2. _____

_____

_____

_____

_____

3. _____

_____

_____

_____

_____

Chapter 10

POSITIVE THINKING

OVERVIEW

This section is devoted to examining how we "talk" to ourselves. We will review some common "thought traps," and you will be encouraged to answer questions that help to counteract irrational thinking.

INTRODUCTION

We all have an "inner voice" that we use to talk to ourselves. This ongoing inner dialogue is a normal part of the way we function, and many of our thoughts and inner questions can be dealt with and then put aside. However, we sometimes have troubling thoughts and questions that cannot easily be laid to rest, and in these cases our inner dialogue can lead to anxiety and stress and can cause negative changes in how we feel and act.

This problem can particularly affect patients with chronic pain. When your pain flares up, you may get stuck on any number of negative thoughts and questions:

- "This pain will make me lose my mind."
- "Soon I may not be able to take care of myself."

- "If it keeps getting worse, how will I manage?"
- "I'm helpless and have no control."
- "No one cares about me."
- "I shouldn't have to hurt."
- "The doctors must have missed something."

Some of my negative thoughts include _____

_____

_____

_____

_____

_____

HOW IRRATIONAL
THOUGHTS ARE BORN

Take time now to complete the Inventory of Negative Thoughts in Response to Pain, at the end of the chapter. This inventory will give you a good idea of the extent to which you have negative thoughts when your pain flares up.

Your mind anticipates problems so that you will be prepared to deal with them. Although this phenomenon, in itself, is not harmful, in anticipating a problem you run the risk of overstating it or of being overly negative about its outcome. Your thoughts about a problematic event - and not necessarily the event itself - are responsible for anxiety, anger, and depression. The diagram on page 104 illustrates how this works.

Clearly, it is important to separate the facts of a situation from your reactions to it. Other "thought traps" that may affect you negatively during a pain flare-up are "catastrophizing" and "absolutizing." To catastrophize means that you come up with the worst possible interpretation of an event. To absolutize means that you tend to think in black-and-white terms. Something is either all bad or all good - there is no middle ground. In either case, you are negatively overreacting to a change and getting stuck with thoughts that are irrational.

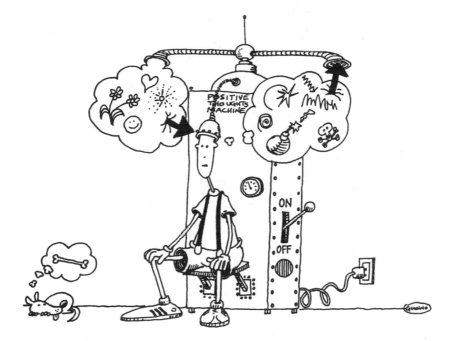

OVERCOMING
IRRATIONAL THOUGHTS

By asking yourself some questions, you can identify thoughts that are irrational or highly improbable:

1. What happened? What led up to the event? Who was there? What did I do? Write down the facts and be objective.
2. How did I perceive the event? Is my perspective in line with everyone else's? (There is a tendency to interpret any event as it affects you. Noting differences between your perspective and that of another person can be helpful in sorting things out.)
3. What were my thoughts about the event? Were my thoughts rational? (A rational idea might be "Muscle spasms are known to accompany chronic pain." An irrational idea might be "I'm going to lose my leg and be totally useless.")

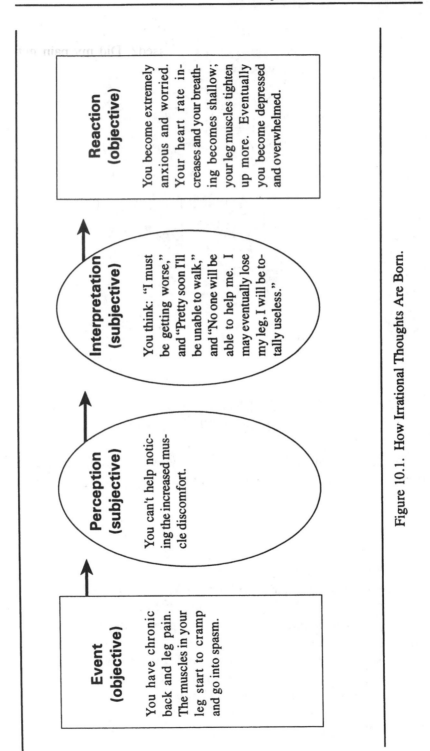

Event (objective)

You have chronic back and leg pain. The muscles in your leg start to cramp and go into spasm.

Perception (subjective)

You can't help noticing the increased muscle discomfort.

Interpretation (subjective)

You think: "I must be getting worse," and "Pretty soon I'll be unable to walk," and "No one will be able to help me. I may eventually lose my leg, I will be totally useless."

Reaction (objective)

You become extremely anxious and worried. Your heart rate increases and your breathing becomes shallow; your leg muscles tighten up more. Eventually you become depressed and overwhelmed.

Figure 10.1. How Irrational Thoughts Are Born.

4. What was my emotional response? Did my thoughts make me feel worthless, angry, or depressed? Did my pain get worse? Did I become more tense and anxious? (Often your thoughts alone can bring on more pain and muscle tension.)

Because irrational thoughts can negatively affect how you feel and act, it is important to question yourself whenever you think that you may be perceiving things irrationally. Some questions to ask are

- Is there any objective support for this idea?
- What evidence exists that this idea is false?
- Does any evidence exist that this idea is true?
- What is the worst thing that could happen to me?
- What good things might happen?

Once you realize that you are having negative irrational thoughts, you need to be able and willing to get yourself "unstuck" by substituting another, more positive thought: "I am going through a bad patch, but I have been able to survive these times in the past." "There are some things I can do to get through this." "This is not a disaster, and I will weather it." "I will be able to manage this pain."

Complete the Inventory of Negative Thoughts in Response to Pain on pages 107 and 108. This will give you an indication of the number and frequency of negative thoughts you have during a flare-up of your pain. If you have had more than 13 of these thoughts you might be prone toward negative thinking.

Inventory of Negative Thoughts
In Response to Pain*

Name: _____

Date: _____

    People who have persistent pain often have flare-ups of their pain. Flare-ups are times when pain increases and is difficult to cope with. These pain flare-ups may last for hours or days.

    During flare-ups people are likely to have a number of negative thoughts. To help us understand your response to pain, we would like to know how often you have different negative thoughts when you experience a flare-up.

    Below is a list of negative thoughts that people have reported having during pain flare-ups. We would like you to read each one, and then check one of the boxes that describe how often you have had that thought during a flare-up of your pain. Check only one box for each thought, and do not skip any items.

	Never	Seldom	Sometimes	Often	Always
SAMPLE: I can't deal with this.	☐	☐	☒	☐	☐
1. I am useless.	☐	☐	☐	☐	☐
2. No one cares about my pain.	☐	☐	☐	☐	☐
3. I've injured myself again.	☐	☐	☐	☐	☐
4. Other people do not believe I have pain.	☐	☐	☐	☐	☐
5. Other people have to do everything for me.	☐	☐	☐	☐	☐
6. My pain is getting worse.	☐	☐	☐	☐	☐

---

*Note: From "The Relationship of Negative Thoughts to Pain and Psychological Distress," by K. Gil, D. A. Williams, F. Keefe, and J. C. Beckham, 1990, *Behavior Therapy, 21*, pp. 349-362. Copyright © 1990 by the Association for Advancement of Behavior Therapy. **Reprinted with permission.**

		Never	Seldom	Sometimes	Often	Always
7.	I can't stand depending on my family and friends anymore.	☐	☐	☐	☐	☐
8.	I cannot control this pain.	☐	☐	☐	☐	☐
9.	It is my own fault I hurt like this.	☐	☐	☐	☐	☐
10.	I am afraid to do anything.	☐	☐	☐	☐	☐
11.	My family has taken over all my responsibilities.	☐	☐	☐	☐	☐
12.	I am going to become an invalid.	☐	☐	☐	☐	☐
13.	I must have done something to bring on this pain.	☐	☐	☐	☐	☐
14.	I am worthless.	☐	☐	☐	☐	☐
15.	No one cares about me anymore.	☐	☐	☐	☐	☐
16.	I can't do anything for others.	☐	☐	☐	☐	☐
17.	I know if I do anything it is going to make my pain worse.	☐	☐	☐	☐	☐
18.	No one wants to hear about my problems.	☐	☐	☐	☐	☐
19.	I can no longer do anything.	☐	☐	☐	☐	☐
20.	It is not fair that I have to live this way.	☐	☐	☐	☐	☐
21.	I am a burden on my family.	☐	☐	☐	☐	☐

22. How often do you have these negative thoughts at times other than during flare-ups (circle one)?

   Never   Seldom   Sometimes   Often   Always

23. To what degree are you able to control these negative thoughts and reduce their frequency (circle one)?

0	1	2	3	4	5	6
No Control			Some Control			Complete Control

The most important points in this chapter that I want to remember are . . .

1. _____

   _____

   _____

   _____

   _____

   _____

2. _____

   _____

   _____

   _____

   _____

   _____

3. _____

   _____

   _____

   _____

   _____

   _____

Chapter 11

PAIN AND DEPRESSION

OVERVIEW

In this chapter you will learn that depression is often associated with chronic pain. A list of ideas is given to help you to break the cycle of depression and pain.

INTRODUCTION

Chronic pain and depression frequently go hand in hand. Feeling depressed about your condition does not mean that you are weak or crazy. In fact, anxiety, fear, sadness, and anger are normal responses to any stressful event in life.

Unfortunately, many patients with chronic pain get into a vicious cycle of pain and depression. Pain that persists for a long time may have consequences such as sleep disturbances, reliance on medication, forced inactivity, and muscle weakness. Because of these difficulties, the person in pain becomes depressed and has negative distorted thoughts and physical reactions. This, in turn, leads to more pain and perpetuates the cycle.

The best way to break this cycle is to make a change in behavior. Unfortunately, most depressed people find it hard to make changes because of the debilitating symptoms of depression, including (a) loss of energy, fatigue, and changes in appetite; (b) loss of sexual interest or pleasure; (c) sleep disturbances; (d) memory and concentration problems; and (e) unhappy moods, including thoughts of suicide.

TYPES OF DEPRESSION

There are two types of depression: endogenous and exogenous. In endogenous depression, there is no precipitating event. Instead, the depression seems to come "out of the blue." In some cases, endogenous depression may be related to chemical reactions within the body. In exogenous or reactive depression, people become depressed in response to loss or stress in their lives.

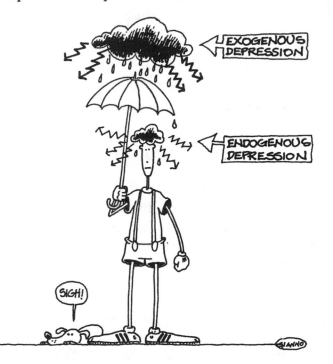

THE LINK BETWEEN
CHRONIC PAIN AND DEPRESSION

Chronic pain leads to depression for a number of reasons. First, fighting pain is exhausting; it tends to sap a great deal of your energy. Thus you must make more of an effort simply to cope with the daily activities that you were able to handle quite easily before your pain began. Second, pain contributes to sleep disturbances. Without proper sleep you can't "recharge" yourself, and you feel physically tired most of the time. Third, chronic pain contributes to worry about failure. Patients often do not know the exact reason for their pain and are concerned about being able to live a productive life in the future. Fourth, most patients with chronic pain have to give up pleasurable events that they have enjoyed in the past. They can no longer travel for long distances or engage in social and recreational activities in the same way as before. All of these difficulties contribute to a loss of self-esteem.

TREATMENT OF DEPRESSION

As part of a pain program, you will be encouraged to make some changes in your behavior to break the cycle of pain and depression. Ways to treat depression related to chronic pain include the following:

1. *Biochemical Treatment.* Some patients with chronic pain apparently have abnormally low levels of serotonin - a substance found in the blood that dilates blood vessels and influences pain. This condition can contribute to sleep problems, increased pain, and depression. Some of these patients take antidepressants which help to alleviate sleep problems and pain intensity.

2. *Exercise and Activity.* Increasing your activity tends to alleviate depression by wearing you out physically and giving you something else to think about. Exercise also appears to increase levels of a chemical in your body (endorphins) that helps to fight pain.

3. *Relaxation.* Using relaxation strategies on a regular basis helps you to cope more effectively with stressful situations and episodes of emotional distress, increasing your energy level and decreasing your depression.

4. *Cognitive Therapy.* Cognitive therapy emphasizes a problem-solving approach to dealing with negative emotions, identifying specific coping behaviors, and altering

negative emotional states. This treatment seeks to change
the way you think about loss, helplessness, failure, and
isolation.

5. *Interpersonal Therapy.* This therapy emphasizes social
relations in treating depression. The treatment focuses on
interpersonal problems you experience when interacting
with others. Emotional expression is encouraged, and
development of new social skills is targeted.

6. *Accomplishment and Success.* By taking a constructive,
active approach to chronic pain and by setting realistic
goals for changing your behavior in ways that will help
you to cope with depression, you can regain a sense of
success and accomplishment. Slow, steady progress translates into long-term success.

☞ **REMEMBER:** *You may have pain, but you do not have
to let the pain have you.*

The most important points in this chapter that I want to remember are . . .

1. _____

   _____

   _____

   _____

   _____

   _____

2. _____

   _____

   _____

   _____

   _____

   _____

3. _____

   _____

   _____

   _____

   _____

   _____

The most important points in this chapter that I wish to remember are:

Chapter 12

PROBLEM SOLVING*

OVERVIEW

This section outlines a problem-solving strategy which you can use to help "objectively" find a solution to any difficulty that you may be experiencing.

INTRODUCTION

This section introduces a stress-management strategy called "SOLVE-Problems." This strategy will help you to identify and evaluate stressful situations and then to consider new ways of behaving in those situations. There are five steps in the SOLVE-Problems strategy:

1. **S**tate the problem.
2. **O**utline the problem.
3. **L**ist possible solutions.
4. **V**iew the consequences.
5. **E**xecute your solution.

---

*Note: This section was adapted with permission from *Self-Management Training Program for Chronic Headache: Patient Manual--Volume II*, by D. B. Penzien and K. A. Holroyd, in press, Sarasota, FL: Professional Resource Press.

Read through the information on the following pages. Then take a look at the sample SOLVE-Problems Worksheet that follows (pp. 123-124).

STEPS FOR SOLVE-PROBLEMS

STEP 1: STATE THE PROBLEM

The first step in solving problems is to identify what they are. It's best if you choose a situation that is often related to your pain. Rate how great a problem it is for you on a scale of 0 to 10, where 0 is "not at all a problem" and 10 is "very much a problem."

STEP 2: OUTLINE THE PROBLEM

Outline the problem on your SOLVE-Problems Worksheet. Include information such as

- Who is involved?
- Where does it happen?
- When does it happen?
- What leads up to it?
- What happens afterward?
- How do you respond?

Thinking about how you respond to a situation is important: Many times you can't change what happens, but often you can change how you respond to what happens. The goal of SOLVE-Problems is to find new and better ways of responding to problem situations.

Outlining the problem may be the most important step in the SOLVE-Problems approach. Accurately describing a problem often helps you to come up with good solutions. Be sure to ask yourself what role you are playing in the problem situation. The point is not to make yourself feel guilty or give yourself a hard time, but to help you to realize that there is a lot you can do to resolve the problem.

STEP 3: LIST POSSIBLE SOLUTIONS

The goal here is to think of many possible solutions. Don't start evaluating any solution before you have finished listing possible options. Getting stuck on one alternative may prevent you from thinking of the best solution. Here are some guidelines to help you generate as many ideas as you can:

1. *Be Creative and Willing to Consider Any Ideas.* Don't be afraid to come up with unlikely or unusual suggestions. At second glance, a solution that seems unlikely may actually be the most likely to succeed.
2. *Quantity Is Best.* The more ideas you generate, the greater the chance that you'll come up with a solution that will work well.
3. *Combine and Refine Your Ideas.* Go back over your list to see if any of your ideas can be grouped together. Sometimes a combination of solutions is your best bet.

STEP 4: VIEW THE CONSEQUENCES

After you have listed the possible solutions, try to come up with at least one positive and one negative consequence for each. Make some notes on these consequences. It may help to ask yourself questions like these:

1. Is this a long-term or a short-term solution? What will happen in the short run if I choose this solution? What will happen in the long run?
2. Will more good come from this solution than harm?
3. How will this solution affect other people?
4. How likely is it that I can actually carry out this solution?
5. How will I feel if I choose this solution? Might I regret it? Will I be proud of myself?
6. Will this solution only partly solve the problem? Will it completely get rid of the problem?

When viewing possible solutions, you should try to be optimistic. One goal of SOLVE-Problems is to encourage you to think of solutions you may not have considered before. Being negative or pessimistic will reduce your chances of finding new solutions.

Some solutions you consider may prove to be too difficult to carry out. Others may be too general to be really useful ("I need to be more assertive with my neighbor"). The best ideas often involve taking small, concrete steps ("I'll ask my neighbor to keep his stereo turned down when I am at home").

When trying to change your behavior, you will benefit from the support of your family and friends. You can talk to them about the changes you are trying to make, ask them to help you generate possible solutions to your problem, or ask them for feedback about a solution you are considering. Knowing that someone you trust agrees with your choice can give you confidence. It's nice to have someone to depend on for help in case everything doesn't work out just right and to have someone with whom to share your accomplishment when things go well.

STEP 5: EXECUTE YOUR SOLUTION

When you're ready, execute your solution. Then write down some notes on how things turned out. Is the problem situation less stressful? Is the problem less likely to cause an increase in pain? How satisfied are you with the outcome? Then rate your problem again, using the same scale you used in Step 1. If you're not satisfied, try going back over Steps 2, 3, and 4, and select a different solution. Then try again.

THE SOLVE-PROBLEMS WORKSHEET

Try to SOLVE at least two of your own problem situations during the upcoming week. When you do the SOLVE-Problems exercise, make sure that you use the worksheet supplied with this manual. When filling out a SOLVE-Problems Worksheet, make sure to

1. *State* the problem. Include your rating of how great a problem the situation is.
2. *Outline* the problem carefully.
3. *List* possible solutions (as many as you can).

4. *View* the consequences, and try to come up with at least one positive and one negative consequence for each solution.

5. *Execute* the best solution. Be sure to write down how well your solution worked.

With practice, this problem-solving strategy will become second nature so that you won't have to write everything down.

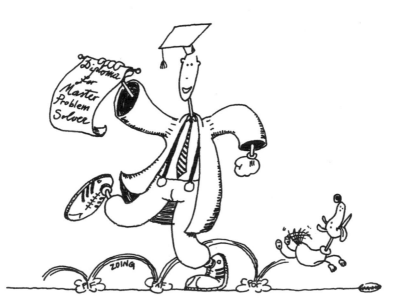

SOLVE-Problems Worksheet

Name: _____ Date: _____

Problem Rating Scale:

0 . . . 1 . . . 2 . . . 3 . . . 4 . . . 5 . . . 6 . . . 7 . . . 8 . . . 9 . . . 10
Not at all   Very much
a problem   a problem

Problem Rating: _____

1. State the problem:

2. Outline the problem:

3. List possible solutions:	4. View the consequences:
a.	a. + -
b.	b. + -

c.	c. + -
d.	d. + -
e.	e. + -
f.	f. + -

5. **Execute your solution:**

_____

Problem Rating After Executing the Solutions: _____

The most important points in this chapter that I want to remember are . . .

1. _____

   _____

   _____

   _____

   _____

   _____

2. _____

   _____

   _____

   _____

   _____

   _____

3. _____

   _____

   _____

   _____

   _____

   _____

Chapter 13

VOCATIONAL REHABILITATION

OVERVIEW

Chronic pain can interfere with your being able to work. This section introduces you to the uses of vocational rehabilitation and to your legal rights with an employer.

INTRODUCTION

When chronic pain affects your ability to work, the consequences can be serious in both economic and psychological terms. More specifically, you may not be able to earn as much money as in the past, and you may feel anxious, fearful, angry, or embarrassed because of your inability to return to work without major adjustments and/or retraining. Vocational rehabilitation can help you get back to work.

ASSESSING YOUR NEED FOR VOCATIONAL REHABILITATION

You need to ask yourself the following questions if most medical treatments for your condition have been tried and you are continuing to have pain:

1. Can I go back to my previous employer and do what I did before?
2. Can I go back to my previous employer and do a different job?
3. Can I go to a different employer and do a job similar to the one I did before?
4. Can I go to a different employer and do a different job?
5. Do I have to be retrained to be able to work again?
6. Is it realistic to think that I will ever be able to work again?

WHAT REHABILITATION COUNSELORS DO

Using your answers to the six questions above as well as information on your personal interests, abilities, limitations, and medical situation, a vocational rehabilitation counselor can help you find appropriate work opportunities. This process may include the following services:

- assessment of aptitudes and interests
- analysis of transferable skills and work potential
- evaluation of physical capacity and work disability
- restorative treatment, such as physical and occupational therapy
- job analysis
- skills training or education
- assessment of employment readiness
- job placement assistance

Together, you and the vocational rehabilitation counselor can develop a plan incorporating both long-range employment goals and the steps that you must take to achieve these goals. As the plan is put into effect, the counselor can meet regularly with you to discuss your progress and help resolve problems that you may encounter. When you are ready to begin work, the counselor can help you find a suitable job and can make contacts to ensure that the placement has been successful.

If you are receiving compensation for a work-related injury, you may be reluctant to return to work for fear that you will be fired if you can't do the job. You need to explore your options so that you can return to work without jeopardizing your benefits. One option might be on-the-job training. Your rehabilitation counselor and a potential employer could set up an agreement under which you would be hired for a limited period (say 3 months). The employer would pay you a minimal wage while you underwent training. You would continue to receive compensation benefits while you found out whether you could do the job. At the end of the training period, the employer would either hire you or write you a letter of recommendation. You would have the option of continuing to receive compensation benefits if you felt that you could not do the job or that the employer was not trust-worthy.

AMERICANS WITH
DISABILITIES ACT (ADA)

The ADA was recently enacted because many individuals with disabilities were discriminated against when they tried to find employment. You may be unsure whether you should let your employer know that you have limitations because you fear either not being hired or being fired. Also, when applying for a job, you may be uncertain whether you should acknowledge that you have received compensation benefits or had a work-related injury.

It is important for you to know your rights. According to the ADA, an employer should make adequate accommodation for your pain-related disability. For instance, you may need to sit in a special chair or to move around periodically. When screening you and making a decision about whether to hire you, an employer cannot ask about disabilities or require a preemployment medical examination. An outline of the main points of the ADA is in Appendix H (pp. 215-216). You may also call your State Reha-bilitation Commission for further information.

Certain companies get a tax advantage by hiring someone with a disability. In this situation, your chronic pain may actually be an advantage. Moreover, educational grants and allowances are available to you if you have a pain-related disability.

Public rehabilitation services are available to all individuals through state agencies. If you were injured on the job and are receiving worker's compensation, your employer may purchase rehabilitation services through a private insurance agency. Anyone denied eligibility for rehabilitation services can appeal the decision to a specified state agency.

BENEFITS OF
REHABILITATION: A SUMMARY

Vocational rehabilitation services can:

1. coordinate services to restore your ability to work and to change your work environment so that the impact of your disability is minimized.
2. help you get retraining for your previous position or a different position at your place of employment.
3. identify suitable vocations and help you enroll in training programs.
4. analyze your job position, work site, and special needs in order to determine what modifications or assistive devices, if any, are required.
5. help you obtain financial compensation or disability benefits to make up for any salary you lose when beginning a new position.
6. inform you of your rights so that you will be able to maintain medical and financial benefits while working.

The most important points in this chapter that I want to remember are . . .

1. _____

_____

_____

_____

_____

_____

2. _____

_____

_____

_____

_____

_____

3. _____

_____

_____

_____

_____

_____

Chapter 14

PAIN AND
SEXUAL ISSUES*

OVERVIEW

This section helps you to understand that pain can contribute to sexual problems. Specific ways are given to help you improve your lovemaking and to gain better control over this common but difficult problem.

INTRODUCTION

A frequent complaint of patients with chronic pain is loss of sexual interest and pleasure. This chapter provides information about the types of problems which may arise and suggests some possible solutions.

For most people, talking about sex is embarrassing. You may have suffered sexual problems in silence because you were embarrassed and thought that nothing could be done. Sexual problems may have interfered with your self-image by causing you to feel less feminine or masculine, less youthful, or less confident socially. It is important to recognize that many people may have problems similar to your own and that your sex life can improve.

---

*Adapted with permission from *Living and Loving: Information About Sex* (pp. 2-6, 8-12), by J. Boggs, 1982, Atlanta, GA: The Arthritis Foundation.

If you have a sexual partner, it may be helpful simply to ask how he or she feels about the way your pain has influenced your sexual activity. Listen to the response. Don't jump to conclusions about what your partner thinks. If your partner's sexual interest seems to have decreased, it may be that he or she is just afraid of causing you pain. Fear of hurting a loved one can short-circuit sexual arousal.

It can be difficult to begin talking about lovemaking. Some partners who joke easily about sex in another setting feel awkward talking about their own sex life. Talking will become easier after you break the ice. You may want to review this chapter with your partner and then talk about the sexual needs, desires, and ideas you both have.

APPROACHING THE PROBLEM

The following ideas may help you get started on improving your lovemaking:

1. *Look Attractive.* Look the best you can every day. Careful grooming will boost your self-image and your morale and will have a positive effect on your interactions with other people.
2. *Be Willing to Talk.* You know what aspects of sexual activity you find comfortable, exciting, or painful. Your partner can know how you feel only if you tell him or her. Words are likely to be clearer than smiles or sighs.
3. *Don't Assume Anything.* Don't assume that your partner feels or thinks the same way you do. Ask what feels good to him or her, and discuss what causes you discomfort and what gives you physical and emotional pleasure.
4. *Develop Your Own Vocabulary.* If you are uncomfortable with words like "penis," "vagina," "clitoris," or "breasts," then use words you both like. Make up some of your own words if that is more comfortable or fun.
5. *Use a Designated Signal.* Agree with your partner on a clear signal to let him or her know that you are experiencing severe pain. A signal can enable you to continue your lovemaking rather than ending it abruptly because of pain or mutual anxiety.

6. *Plan Ahead.* Plan to engage in sexual activity at the time of day when you generally feel best. If you use medication to manage your pain, time the dose to minimize your pain during intercourse.
7. *Pace Yourself.* Pacing all your activities during the day will keep you from being too tired to enjoy making love. You should also pace yourself during your lovemaking activity.
8. *Relax Ahead of Time.* Using relaxation techniques before making love may help to decrease worry and tension. A warm bath or shower before sex may also be relaxing and soothing.
9. *Share Your Experience.* Always let your mate know when something really feels good.

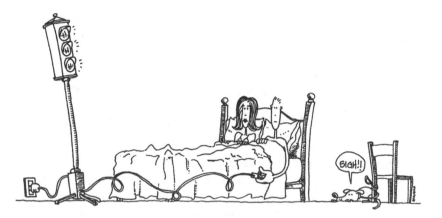

CHOOSING A POSITION

The position you choose for intercourse can help or hinder your sex life. For example, one common position - with the woman on her back and the man over her - can be very uncomfortable if either partner is experiencing low-back or joint pain. Think about what positions you assume to make yourself more comfortable when you are simply lying in bed, and then try to adapt these positions for lovemaking. Along with position, consider what types of movements during sex increase your pain; one partner may need to do most of the moving.

The following descriptions of lovemaking positions are just suggestions. Since people differ in height, weight, strength, and degree of pain, each couple will need to accommodate to specific needs.

Position 1: Both partners lie on their side, with the woman facing away from the man. The man enters from behind. The woman can have a pillow between her knees. This position is helpful when the woman has back and hip pain.

Position 2: The woman lies on her back, with a pillow under her hips and thighs. The male partner lies on top of her while supporting his weight with his hands and knees. This position is useful when the woman has back, hip, or lower-extremity pain.

Position 3: Both partners lie on their side, facing each other. This position is recommended when the man has low-back pain because the woman provides most of the hip movement.

Position 4: Both partners are standing. The man enters from behind. The woman may use furniture at a comfortable height for support and balance. The woman may also kneel, with her knees and upper body supported.

Position 5: The man lies on his back. He may use a pillow for support. The woman sits on top of the man, supporting her weight with her hands and knees. This position is used when the man has back, hip, or knee pain and requires that the woman provide most of the movement.

CONSIDERING ALTERNATIVES

There are a number of alternative ways to make love. All are normal and natural expressions of human sexuality. These options may be welcome during painful episodes. For example, manual sex, with fondling and stroking of the genitals, the breasts, or other areas of sensitivity, can offer a fulfillment as complete as that obtained from intercourse. The use of a vibrator or oral sex may also be fulfilling. Your exploration of alternatives to intercourse should begin with mutual agreement and continue with patience and consideration. Whatever options you choose, your warmth, caring, and reassuring embrace can convey your love fully.

Despite your best efforts, there may be times when you do not become sexually aroused. At these times you can still provide for the needs of your partner by using alternative methods just described. A particular concern for men is the inability to get an erection. As a man learns about what a woman enjoys, he will become more confident that he can bring her pleasure and fulfillment without an erection. His feeling of masculinity may even be heightened through expanding sexual experience, and his returning confidence may eventually restore his ability to get an erection.

GETTING HELP

Should emotional complications arise between you and your partner, such as resentment, guilt, or any other strong negative feelings related to your physical relationship, counseling can be useful. Do not hesitate to share your concerns with a therapist or counselor. Reading material can be made available to give you further information.

The most important points in this chapter that I want to remember are . . .

1. _____

   _____

   _____

   _____

   _____

   _____

2. _____

   _____

   _____

   _____

   _____

   _____

3. _____

   _____

   _____

   _____

   _____

   _____

Chapter 15

WEIGHT MANAGEMENT
AND NUTRITION

OVERVIEW

This chapter offers information on why persons with chronic pain often have weight management problems and what steps can be taken to help.

INTRODUCTION

One common side effect of chronic pain is weight gain. Many physicians and health professionals simply tell patients with chronic pain to "lose some weight and you will feel better." There is no evidence that weight loss will make chronic pain go away. It is true, however, that you will feel more in control and have a better self-image if you keep yourself at a good weight. If you have chronic pain, it may be very difficult to lose weight even though you eat very little. Since movement can make chronic pain worse, you may tend to avoid exercise. Unfortunately, in the long run, a lack of exercise can actually increase your pain by contributing to such problems as emotional distress and immobility of the joints. The nutritional deficiencies resulting from poor eating habits can also make your pain worse.

141

FACTORS IN
WEIGHT-CONTROL PROBLEMS

As a chronic pain patient, you may have trouble losing weight for a number of reasons. First, you may tend to be inactive. The formula is simple: intake = output + storage; or, put another way, food = activity + fat. If you stop exercising, your metabolic rate slows down. A slower metabolic rate means that fewer calories are burned and that food is more likely to be converted into fat.

Second, with inactivity you replace muscle tissue with fat. Having less muscle means you tend to burn fewer calories.

Third, dieting can actually backfire. A very low-calorie diet without exercise can fool your body into thinking it is starving. Your metabolic rate slows down, and you tend not to burn up stored energy (fat).

Fourth, you may have an increased desire to eat highly fattening foods. Some researchers believe that this craving is related to the loss of certain substances in response to chronic pain.

Finally, chronic pain tends to interfere with many of the things that you enjoyed doing in the past. One way to substitute for your loss of other forms of enjoyment is to eat.

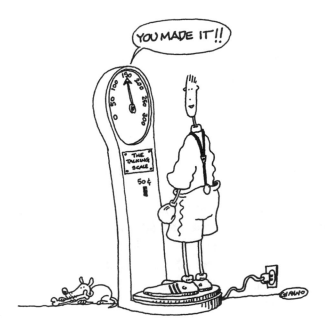

TIPS FOR
WEIGHT MANAGEMENT

1. *Increase Your Level of Exercise.* Sticking to a schedule of regular exercise can be hard. However, exercise can contribute significantly to weight loss - perhaps even more significantly than what you eat.

2. *Eat Less Fat, Sugar, and Processed Food.* Examples include butter, fried foods, fast foods, and fatty meats.

3. *Eat More Complex Carbohydrates, Vegetables, Lean Meats, and Fruit.* Examples include whole-grain bread, baked (not fried) potatoes, baked chicken, low-fat ham and turkey, steamed vegetables, and fresh fruit.

4. *Watch Your Snacks.* Most snack foods are high in fat. When in doubt, read the label on the package to find out how much fat, protein, and carbohydrate each snack has. For example, potato chips are 60% fat, while pretzels are only 15% fat.

5. *Drink Lots of Water.* During the summer you may want to drink up to eight full glasses of water a day. Drinking large amounts of water fills you up and suppresses your appetite.

6. *Don't Let Yourself Get Too Hungry.* Four small meals of 500 calories each will probably feel more satisfying than two meals of 1,000 calories each. Also, moderate snacking throughout the day on low-fat foods such as pretzels will help prevent overeating at mealtimes.

7. *Keep a Record of Your Progress.* Keep a food, exercise, and weight diary to help you assess how you're doing and what you need to change. Begin by completing the Daily Food Diary on pages 211-212.

8. *Eat Slowly.* Since it takes time for food to be absorbed into your system, rapid eating may prevent you from feeling satisfied until you have eaten more than you need to.

9. *Plan Ahead.* Avoiding last-minute decisions about food can prevent impulsive eating. You may want to prepare your food in the morning, label it according to the time you will eat it, then put it in a special place. When you do your food shopping, go to the store with a full stomach and stick to a list.

10. *Take a Hunger Check.* Before you eat a meal or a snack, ask yourself whether you are really hungry. If not, delay your meal or have a snack that is low in calories.

11. *Overcome "Emotional" Eating.* Chronic pain patients frequently report eating when they feel angry, bored, or depressed. Use some of the problem-solving strategies in this book to avoid this kind of eating. (See Chapters 11 and 12.)

12. *Check Your Medication.* Ask your physician whether any medication that you are presently taking tends to contribute to weight gain. Some medications for pain, in particular tricyclic antidepressants, have weight gain as a side effect. Also, remember that alcohol is high in calories and stimulates hunger.

13. *Be Patient.* In trying to gain self-control, it is easy to become discouraged. Everyone has periodic setbacks. Take things one step at a time, work for short-term goals, and congratulate yourself on small achievements. Remember that weight loss is less important than weight maintenance.

14. *Try to Stick to the Following Guidelines:*

- Use smaller plates.
- Leave food on your plate.
- Serve yourself more than once, using smaller portions.
- While cooking, keep snack foods out of sight.
- Throw away any food left on your plate immediately after the meal.
- Have only one designated eating place, and allow yourself to eat only at that place.
- Do not do any other activities while you are eating.
- Keep serving platters and containers off the table.
- Avoid accepting food from other people unless you have asked for it.

Refer to these guidelines when completing your Individual Weight Management Goal Sheet on page 145.

If you need additional information about weight management, consult with a nutritionist, psychologist, or physician. A lot of information is available to help you lose and maintain you weight.

Individual Weight
Management Goal Sheet

Date: _____

1. My goal for weight change for the coming _____ week(s)
    is _____ pound(s).
2. The following are my goals for eating habits for the coming week
    (Please remember to keep standards specific and objective - i.e., "I
    will have a snack only once per week between meals" is specific
    and objective. "I will try to do better on snacking" is not.):

EATING HABIT GOALS

1. _____

    _____

    _____

    _____

2. _____

    _____

    _____

    _____

3. _____

    _____

    _____

    _____

4. _____

    _____

    _____

    _____

5. _____

    _____

    _____

    _____

The most important points in this chapter that I want to remember are . . .

1. _____

   _____

   _____

   _____

   _____

   _____

2. _____

   _____

   _____

   _____

   _____

   _____

3. _____

   _____

   _____

   _____

   _____

   _____

Chapter 16

PROBLEMS WITH MEMORY
AND CONCENTRATION

OVERVIEW

In this section we will review some problems that persons with chronic pain may have with memory and concentration and will list some strategies that you can use to improve your memory.

INTRODUCTION

Many people with chronic pain report problems with their ability to remember and concentrate. The most likely explanation for these difficulties is simply that the pain interferes with the ability to store and recall information. As a person with chronic pain, you may sometimes find yourself unable to concentrate well enough to read, watch television, or complete a task; if you are going through vocational rehabilitation, your problems with concentration may be interfering with your ability to learn new skills required for a job. You may frequently misplace things you need or forget something that you have read or watched within a short time. Although these problems can lower your self-confidence and cause complications in your daily life, you can minimize their impact by using a variety of strategies to improve your memory and concentration.

DEALING WITH
MEMORY PROBLEMS

Here are some ideas for improving your memory and concentration:

1. *Notice Your Memory Problems.* Identify instances in which you have had problems with memory and concentration in the past, and use this information to predict problems you may have in the future. Notice the times at which your memory and concentration are relatively good and the times at which they are poor.

2. *Reduce Outside Interference.* Distractions contribute to memory problems. Try to pay attention to only one thing at a time, and recognize that overly stimulating circumstances can drastically reduce your ability to remember and concentrate.

3. *Write It Down.* Make notes to yourself. Use "Post-it" notes around the house to jog your memory. Since something is easier to remember when it is associated with a particular action, the act of making a note will help regardless of whether you consult your notes later.

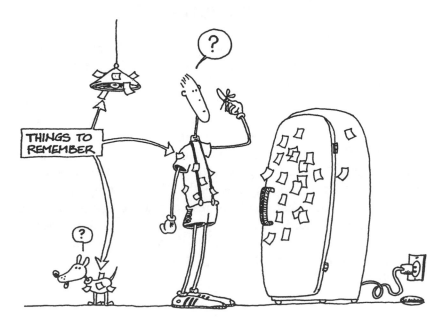

4. *Create Memory Associations.* Link the thing you want to remember with one of your regular activities or with something that you routinely do remember. You can use any repetitive action, such as looking at your watch or brushing your teeth, to remember something else you need to do.

5. *Use Relaxation.* When you are most tense and anxious, it is most difficult to recall information. Relaxation strategies can be helpful in this regard.

6. *Create an Image.* Some people use imagery to improve memory. You can form a mental picture of something you need to remember, or you can associate things that you need to remember (such as items on a shopping list) with other articles in you home.

7. *Repeat Things Out Loud.* By reciting something out loud, you use two functions - speech and hearing - to increase your chances of remembering it. Also, stating what you need to remember in your own words helps you to "own" the information.

8. *Review What You Have Learned.* One way to transfer information from your short-term memory to your long-term memory is to review what you want to remember after several minutes or hours. The more you review information, the more likely you'll be to remember it.

9. *Examine Any Irrational Thoughts.* Some individuals tend to catastrophize their situation, worrying that their mental faculties are rapidly deteriorating. Avoid negative and self-blaming thoughts, such as "I have no mind anymore" or "I can't remember anything." Instead, reassure yourself that persons with chronic pain frequently have problems with memory and concentration and that tricks and strategies can be used to help improve these capabilities.

10. *Create and Use Mnemonics.* A mnemonic is a trick used to remember something. An example is to create a word out of the first letter of each of a list of words you want to remember, such as the items on the shopping list you've accidentally left at home. It will take some creativity and practice on your part but can be a powerful tool. An example used in this manual is the acronym SOLVE. This stands for state the problem (S), outline the problem (O),

list the solutions (L), view the consequences (V), and
execute (E).

Using a combination of these techniques should help you to
improve your memory. You may also want to consult some of the
many self-help books on memory improvement.

The most important points in this chapter that I want to remember are . . .

1. _____

_____

_____

_____

_____

_____

2. _____

_____

_____

_____

_____

_____

3. _____

_____

_____

_____

_____

_____

Chapter 17

HUMOR, HAPPINESS, AND PAIN

OVERVIEW

This chapter discusses the unhappiness you may be experiencing as a result of your pain and what you can do about it. It offers a number of specific tips on changing your behavior and outlook in ways that may make you a happier person again.

MEANING OF HAPPINESS

Happiness and pain are two words that are rarely heard together: People who continually hurt are not generally thought of as happy. Much of your unhappiness may stem from pain, and the losses that may have accompanied it: loss of activity, loss of income, loss of social life, loss of self-confidence, loss of fulfillment, and loss of purpose in life. Friends and family members may try to offer encouragement by saying that "there are people who are worse off than you." This does not make your situation any better and can lead to considerable anger that others do not understand how disastrous your condition has been for you. Yet, despite all of the problems associated with pain, some pain sufferers are able to say that they are happy. When asked to elaborate, they often say that they have gained an appreciation for the positive "little" things and don't let negative things get to them. Most

155

of the research on happiness suggests that people who are happy
are very aware of ordinary events and take great pleasure in small
achievements.   People who are generally unhappy often have
thoughts about what they do not have rather than what they do
have.   Individuals who are happy greatly appreciate what they
have. It is of little help to you to minimize what has happened.
However, *happiness is a state of mind that you can cultivate* by
examining your thoughts, feelings, and behaviors.

Norman Cousins, who was diagnosed with a painful degenerative condition and wrote of his experience in *Anatomy of Illness*
(1979 [New York: Bantam Books]), found a way to minimize his
debilitating pain by using laughter in his daily routine. He sought
out jokes, movies, and books which would contribute to a daily
"belly laugh." He found that a good laugh eased his pain for up
to a half an hour. The goal was not to "laugh off" his pain but
rather to achieve a physical state which would relieve it.

There is evidence that laughter leads to a number of physical
reactions that actually decrease pain.   These include decreased
production of stress associated hormones, relaxation of muscle
groups, slowed breathing, and increased circulation. Watching a
funny movie produces these physical changes in us. Studies have
demonstrated that humor can decrease fatigue, anxiety, and depression, and helps to combat pain.

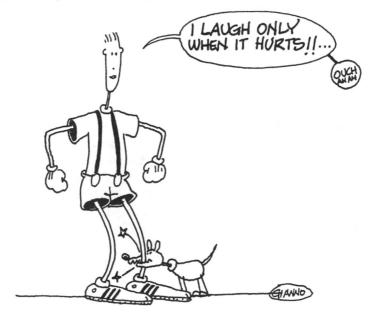

SEARCH FOR HAPPINESS

The following are some suggestions for improving your mood and outlook on life:

1. *Set Realistic Goals to Gradually Improve Your Sense of Well-Being.* Happiness can be learned. There are things you can do on purpose to improve your outlook. Start by making a commitment to yourself that you will change your perspective and work to be happier.

2. *Try Not to Compare Yourself Now With the Way You Were Before.* Our judgment of whether something is good or bad is often related to what we compare it to. For example, you can get upset if you think you paid too much for something, while, getting a "bargain" makes you feel good. In fact, your feelings are related to your comparisons of a situation with some other situation. In the same way, you can get upset when you think about all that you have lost because of your pain. Unfortunately, dwelling on what you have lost guarantees that you will feel unhappy and discontented.

3. *Use Humor Whenever Possible.* By seeking out humor in everyday situations you may be able to put some distance between yourself and your pain. Humor can help to make your situation appear much less dismal. Each day, set a goal for yourself to tell a good story that will make someone else laugh.

4. *Socialize With Others* (even though you don't feel like it). Isolating yourself from others often does not improve your mood. By acting as if things are OK, and keeping your mind occupied while you are around other people, you have a better chance of improving your mood. Try to especially seek out those who share your same sense of humor, and avoid those who are bound to make you depressed.

5. *Smile and Act Happy.* Researchers have shown that simply acting as if you are happy can ultimately change your perception of yourself and the perception others have about you. Even though others may suspect that all is not well, acting as if you were in a good mood and managing well

may ultimately have a positive effect on how you see
yourself and your situation.

6. *Seek Sensual Pleasure.*   Most people with chronic pain
    have little to look forward to throughout the day. Chronic
    pain tends to cancel out any pleasures which you may
    experience. It is important, however, to schedule some
    time to do things that may calm you and offer some pleas-
    ure. For example, you may choose to spend time listening
    to good music, enjoying a certain food, viewing an attrac-
    tive landscape, or using comfort measures for your pain.

7. *Pursue Those Things Which Are Most Exciting to You.*
    Even though pain has a way of restricting your activities
    and interfering with your memory and concentration, pursu-
    ing hobbies and vocations that are exciting to you is very
    important. You may want to learn to be a gourmet cook,
    or learn how to repair a lock. By becoming successful at
    something that interests you, you will become more self-
    confident.

8. *Use Confirming Self-Statements.*   People who are happy
    tend to keep positive thoughts in the back of their mind:
    "I am a good person." "I have a purpose." "I am in con-
    trol." "I have a lot of good qualities." "I am important."
    Research suggests that regardless of whether you believe
    that these totally apply to you, repeating them to yourself
    can help to change your perception of yourself.

9. *Apply Flexible Thinking.* Seeing things as either "black or
    white" can make you unhappier than you have to be when
    things are not going well. Things are rarely all bad or all
    good. You need to be open to different ways of looking at
    things. A stiff tree is more likely to fall in a hurricane
    than a flexible one. You need to reorganize the way that
    you perceive yourself and others in order to accept the
    many changes that have happened to you.

10. *Create a List of "One Liners" to Those Questions You
    Hate.* Part of the reason that people with pain shy away
    from social events is that well-meaning people ask many
    questions that you are tired of answering: Is your pain any
    better? Isn't there something that your doctor can do?
    When are you going to get better? Can't they just go in
    and fix it? How come you don't look like you are hurting?

Develop a set of one liners for friends and relatives who offer the same advice every time that you see them: "Oh, I only limp to get your attention." "My doctors love to see me so much that they have all secretly decided not to make me better." "I am doing penance for my past lives." "My pain is doing better each day - the more I hurt the better my pain is doing."

11. *Change Your Posture So That You Look Alive and Happy.* People who are depressed often tend to slump their shoulders, hang their head, and look tired and exhausted. By standing up as straight as possible, smiling, and walking tall, you can positively affect your mood.

12. *Run a Movie in Your Mind.* Some individuals can make themselves feel good by recalling past events which were very enjoyable. Playing these memorable events or occasions over in your mind can lift your spirits. Your imagination is a very powerful tool in combating stressful thoughts.

13. *Keep Hoping That Things Will Get Better.* People who manage well with their pain tend to remain optimistic despite ups and downs. They maintain positive thoughts and a strong belief that their condition will improve with time. Belief that there is a positive purpose to everything that happens to you will improve your ability to cope and give you daily strength and encouragement.

The most important points in this chapter that I want to remember are . . .

1. _____

_____

_____

_____

_____

_____

2. _____

_____

_____

_____

_____

_____

3. _____

_____

_____

_____

_____

_____

Chapter 18

HOW TO BE "SMART"
ABOUT YOUR PAIN

OVERVIEW

This chapter offers some common-sense advice on helping you to cope intelligently with your pain.

INTRODUCTION

Being "smart" about your pain means changing your behavior in ways that help you cope with your situation. You may not be able to do everything the way you used to do it before. In the past, for example, if you started a job you may have kept at it until it was done; now you may need to do the job in stages over a longer period. You may have had certain standards about how your house should be kept or how active you should be; those standards may not be practical now. Although changing your behavior is hard, it's the smart response.

Here are some tips on how to be smart about your pain:

1. *Work Toward Control.* Aim at being in control of your condition more than 50% of the time.
2. *Be Prepared.* Anticipate what may happen to you in a given situation. If you are asked to go somewhere or do something, think about it. Ask yourself questions like the

following: Will I be standing, sitting, or walking? What will the seats be like? How many people will be there? Will I be able to leave or lie down if I have to? Will I be able to talk openly to the person I am with? What will be expected of me?

3. *Decide and Stick to Your Decision.* When the day of a particular event or activity comes, decide whether you should participate. If you're having a bad day, you will need to avoid any activity that will throw your pain out of control. Although it's not easy, you must listen to yourself and be firm about your decision. Don't be talked into doing something that you know you will regret later.

4. *Decide to Hurt.* Sometimes you may choose to do something that you want to do even though you know it will make your pain worse. As long as you think it through and recognize what the consequences will be, this decision is all right.

5. *Have a Plan for Dealing With Your Pain.* If you decide to do something that will make your pain worse, have a plan for your recovery afterward. What type of treatment will you use? How easy will it be for you to get some rest? How will you pace your activities? What will you have to give up?

6. *Pick an Alternate Activity.* If you decide not to undertake a certain activity, figure out something to do instead. The worst thing you can do is to stay home doing nothing and feeling angry, depressed, and guilty about your choices.

7. *Take One Moment at a Time.* Remind yourself to take things one hour or one day at a time. Worrying about the future probably will not be productive and may lead to more anxiety and pain. Catch yourself on those occasions when you are most upset and worried. Are you dealing with the present, or are you thinking into the future and anticipating the worst?

8. *Don't Dwell on What You Cannot Change.* Try to figure out which things are out of your control, and then try not to worry about them. You cannot undo what has happened to you, but you can control how you react to it.

9. *Cooperate Rather Than Collide.* At times, chronic pain can dictate your life and destroy your peace of mind. You

may tend to resist your pain for fear of giving in to it. The truth is that you need to reach some understanding of yourself and your condition. This is a sign not of weakness but of strength. Working toward acceptance of the conditions of your day-to-day existence may help restore your peace of mind.

10. *Remember the 3 P's:*

- **P**ick what you can do.
- **P**lan what you do.
- **P**repare for what will happen.

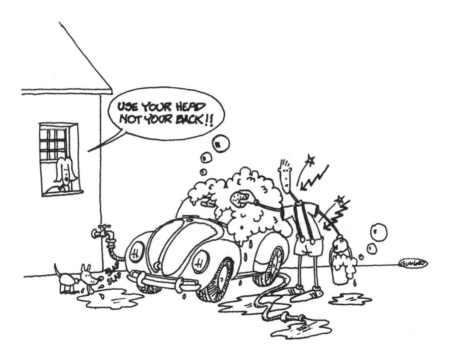

Here are the ways that I choose to be smarter about my pain . . .

1. _____

_____

_____

_____

_____

2. _____

_____

_____

_____

_____

3. _____

_____

_____

_____

_____

Chapter 19

HOW TO GET
THE MOST HELP FROM
THE MEDICAL SYSTEM

OVERVIEW

*Persons with chronic pain see many health profession-
als for help with their condition. This section discusses some ways that you can get the most benefit
from these professionals.*

INTRODUCTION

Individuals with chronic medical problems have to deal with
a complicated and sometimes overly bureaucratic medical system.
Today doctors tend to specialize in particular areas of medicine.
People with chronic pain often see a variety of specialists (inter-
nists, orthopedists, neurologists, neurosurgeons, anesthesiologists,
rheumatologists, psychiatrists) as well as other health care professionals (psychologists, social workers, physical therapists, acu-
puncturists, chiropractors). Each of these individuals may have a
different slant on your diagnosis and make a different recommendation for treatment. After being seen by many specialists, you
may end up with the same amount of pain you began with, and
you may feel confused about who is responsible for your care. In

169

addition, your dealings with employers, insurance carriers, and lawyers may cause you to feel trapped by a system that is time-consuming, complex, and frustrating.

If you gain a better understanding of the medical system, you will receive better treatment for your condition. The following points are worth considering:

1. *Learn Which Providers Can Be Most Helpful.* Some doctors and health care professionals who genuinely want to help you may not be able to do so because their training and expertise aren't relevant to your problem. These doctors may have trouble telling you that they don't know what to do; instead, after they have exhausted their treatment options, they may ask you to come back in 6 months or a year, or they may refer you elsewhere. You should consult other persons in pain to find out which doctors have been helpful to them; try to figure out early on whether you think the doctor you are seeing can be helpful, and don't take it personally if you are referred elsewhere.

2. *Strive to be Understood.* Chronic pain is a confusing condition to have, and it is also confusing to treat. Some doctors may have trouble totally understanding what is causing your problem. Be consistent, honest, and clear in communicating with your doctor, and try not to be defensive if you aren't immediately understood. Don't hesitate to try again and to stand up for yourself - as firmly and calmly as you can - if you feel you aren't being heard.

3. *Build Trust.* Once you have found a doctor you feel can be most helpful to you, do all you can to get to know him or her and to build trust. Particularly if the doctor is prescribing medication that can be abused, he or she needs to know that you have good judgment and a strong sense of responsibility. Being calm, straight-forward, and friendly will help.

4. *Make the Best Use of Your Doctor's Time.* Doctors are under constant time pressure and appreciate your coming prepared for your appointments. Write down your questions in advance and bring along any information you have that may help your doctor understand your problem. Avoid

turning your chronic pain into an emergency; specifically, don't habitually wait until you are in a crisis to phone your doctor with urgent demands for immediate attention.

5. *Get to Know the People Involved in Your Treatment.* If the receptionists, nurses, and doctors involved get to know you as a pleasant, reasonable person, you will stand a better chance of getting prompt help when you really need it.

6. *Work Within the System.* Find out from employees or other patients how your doctor's office or clinic is set up and then follow the standard procedures. If you don't, you may create problems and/or end up not getting the best treatment, even if everyone has the best intentions.

7. *Use Your Pain Management Tools.* By using the pain management techniques discussed in this manual, you can become an "adaptive coper" and improve your chances of getting helpful treatment. Regularly using relaxation, pacing, rational thinking, and problem-solving strategies can increase your control of your problem and make you an easier patient to work with and treat.

Although we live in a society that offers the most advanced medical services in the world, the treatment of chronic pain is not an exact science. Much depends on your understanding of the problem, your active participation in dealing with it, and your relationships with health care professionals. By becoming a knowledgeable consumer, you can get the most from the medical system.

The most important points in this chapter that I want to remember are . . .

1. _____

_____

_____

_____

_____

_____

2. _____

_____

_____

_____

_____

_____

3. _____

_____

_____

_____

_____

_____

Chapter 20

SOCIAL SUPPORT SYSTEMS

OVERVIEW

This chapter briefly discusses the importance of support in managing your pain. It reviews support issues as they relate to you, your family, your community, and your friends. You will be asked to complete questions about your support system and to look at ways of improving it.

SUPPORT: GOOD OR BAD?

Your social support system consists of one person or a number of people who reliably help meet your emotional needs. These individuals reinforce your sense of self-worth, provide you with valuable feedback about yourself, and offer help during a crisis. Your social support network can include family, friends, neighbors, and contacts you have made in religious groups or social clubs.

Chronic pain can erode your social support just when you may need it the most. Chronic pain is not just a one-person problem; it affects everyone around you. You may have little desire to interact with others or to participate in social or recreational events. Eventually you may have fewer and fewer people around who can be supportive. Since you are not able to do as much as you used to, you may not have the chance to return favors to those who help you. As a result, you may tend not to ask for help. In these situations, support from others may actually make you feel worse.

Nevertheless, social support is very important in dealing with chronic pain. People who seem to manage well with their pain often come from families who are supportive, creative, and flexible. Those who perceive their families and friends as being highly supportive often report less anxiety, depression, and irritability; a better quality of life; and greater benefit from treatment. Support from other people can serve to distract you and can pull you out of a depression. Evidence suggests that a solid social network helps buffer stress, prevents further health problems, and makes harmful or threatening experiences less worrisome. In short, support can help you cope with your pain.

If you feel that you have had only limited support in dealing with your persistent pain, you are not alone. People with pain frequently encounter a number of family, community, and spiritual support issues related to their pain.

FAMILY SUPPORT ISSUES

Chronic pain can have a negative impact on your marital relationship and lead to strained interactions with children and other relatives. Your sex life may deteriorate, and you may feel a loss of intimacy. Your pain can change the roles played by everyone in the family, causing tension, frustration, and guilt. Spouses and other family members may even make your condition worse out of their concern for you. For example, they may keep you from doing things for yourself and limiting your activities. By taking on many of the jobs which you used to perform, they may leave you feeling useless and unimportant. Your pain may also influence communication patterns in the family. You may have been left out of important conversations in an effort not to hurt your feelings.

COMMUNITY SUPPORT ISSUES

Pain often keeps you from engaging in activities in which you would normally participate. If you have been out of work because of your pain, you may have less contact with other people than you would have if you were working. Pain can change your interaction with former co-workers and social contacts. You may feel uncomfortable because other people do not understand what you have been going through or because they continue to be involved in activities that you no longer participate in. Membership in social groups can be especially difficult because of your limited ability to participate. The unpredictability of your pain may be such that other members will not be able to rely on you to undertake projects and assume responsibilities like you had done in the past.

SPIRITUAL SUPPORT ISSUES

Some individuals with chronic pain feel isolated regardless of whether there are supportive people around them. They may feel empty and wonder whether life is worth living. No matter what your religious beliefs, we all have spiritual needs. These needs often remain below the surface until disaster strikes. When you are in pain, many spiritual questions may arise. These are difficult questions to answer. The following questions are frequently raised by persons with chronic pain:

- Why do I have to suffer?
- Am I being punished?
- How can I make sense of what has happened to me?
- How can I still be useful to and needed by others?
- Has my life been worthless?
- Is it my fault that I am like this?
- Why does God allow me to suffer like this?
- Why do bad things happen in the world, especially to good people?

A church or synagogue can provide knowledgeable professionals who can discuss these questions with you, provide attention to your spiritual needs, and offer a support system which can help to combat your loneliness.

WHAT CAN BE DONE TO
IMPROVE YOUR SUPPORT

Take the time to complete the Social Support Questionnaire at the end of this chapter (pp. 181-183). Add up your score and use it as a way to determine how you perceive your support system.

Although "perceived support" is an important ingredient in your ability to cope with your pain, it can be difficult to make changes that improve your social support network. If you have found it difficult to maintain close community and social ties, you can improve your situation. You can also assess your spiritual needs and find some peace within yourself. The following points are worth considering:

1. *Recognize That Pain Can Make You Feel Abandoned (Even by God).* Chronic pain not only influences your physical capacity to remain active but also contributes to your emotional isolation. It is common for individuals with chronic pain to feel isolated and alone. It is important to know that many people experience this sense of isolation when they are in chronic pain.

2. *We All Have Social and Spiritual Needs.* We are social beings who need to interact with others and to explore our spiritual concerns. It is unnatural for humans to hide themselves away from all contact with others or to ignore the spiritual side of themselves.

3. *No One Has a Satisfactory Answer to Questions About Suffering.* From the beginning of humankind we have been trying to explain why bad things happen. People with chronic pain often report feelings of guilt, as if they are being punished for something they might have done. These feelings are normal, and questions about suffering should be openly discussed.

4. *Talking Can Help.* It is important to share your feelings with others. You may find that certain family members are too close to the problem to be able to listen to all of your worries and concerns. It is important to seek out people who can address your feelings of isolation and abandonment. These people may include therapists, counselors, clergy, social service providers, and so on.

5. *Prayer Can Help.* Prayer is a powerful way to receive personal comfort. It may seem at times that your prayers have not been answered. It is also very difficult to pray when your beliefs have been put to the test. But the act of praying has been shown to increase feelings of well-being. Reading Psalms from the Bible is a way to gain perspective and obtain a sense of peace when you feel confused. Consult owners of religious bookstores about reading materials that offer comfort and direction.

6. *Make an Effort to Change Your Social Support System.* Maintaining contacts with friends that you have known in the past may make you feel awkward and uncomfortable. Determine who can be most helpful to you and seek them out. Do not force yourself to maintain relationships that have dramatically changed since the onset of your pain. You may be in a different place and no longer share the things that you once had in common.

7. *Inquire About Pain Support Groups.* There are a number of organizations that offer support to those with chronic pain. Consult your physician, local hospital, newspaper, or directory for information on what might be available to you. Avoid those groups where much of the conversation is focused on negative topics. Seek out a group with a facilitator who will lead the discussion in a positive direction and limit the "moan and groan" elements. If you have a computer and modem, you might consider conversing with others through the Internet, Prodigy, America OnLine, Compuserve, or another interactive computer network program.

8. *Tell Yourself You Have Something to Offer.* There is a tendency to be "your own worst enemy" when you are in pain. It is hard to recognize that you are valuable and important to others. Resist thoughts that you are no longer

useful because of what you cannot do, and recognize that you can be valuable for just being you.

9. *See Your Physician as a Source of Support.* Many health care professionals can be very helpful in getting you through a difficult time. You may have overlooked asking your doctor for help. You may be surprised at how willing he or she may be to listen to you and offer concrete suggestions.

10. *Miracles Happen When Your Outlook Changes.* People with chronic pain often hope that a miracle will happen and their pain will disappear forever. Unfortunately for many, an instant cure does not happen. Much of the emotional distress that people with chronic pain experience is related to their perception of themselves and what has happened to them. A change in perception often leads to less distress, improved coping, and a greater sense of control. Patients completing a pain program often report that their adjustment to their pain has improved. They come to achieve a positive yet realistic outlook about their condition. These results may well be seen as a miracle!

Social Support Questionnaire*

Directions: This is a questionnaire used to measure your perceived support. Answer each question as honestly as possible and then follow the directions at the end to obtain your overall score.

1. When you are in pain, how often is your husband/wife/other family member supportive and encouraging?

1	2	3	4	5	6	7	8	9	10
Never		Seldom		Sometimes			Frequently		Always

2. When you are in pain, how often does your husband/wife/other family member ignore you or become angry with you?

1	2	3	4	5	6	7	8	9	10
Never		Seldom		Sometimes			Frequently		Always

3. When you are in pain, how often do you feel a loss of spiritual support?

1	2	3	4	5	6	7	8	9	10
Never		Seldom		Sometimes			Frequently		Always

4. How satisfied are you with the support you have from your family?

1	2	3	4	5	6	7	8	9	10
Very Dissatisfied		Fairly Dissatisfied		A Little Dissatisfied		A Little Satisfied		Fairly Satisfied	Very Satisfied

5. How satisfied are you with the support you have from your friends and social community?

1	2	3	4	5	6	7	8	9	10
Very Dissatisfied		Fairly Dissatisfied		A Little Dissatisfied		A Little Satisfied		Fairly Satisfied	Very Satisfied

---

*Adapted with permission from *Social Support Measure*, by K. Gil and T. R. Kinney, 1989, Durham, NC: Duke University Medical Center.

6. How satisfied are you with the support you receive through your spiritual convictions?

1	2	3	4	5	6	7	8	9	10
Very Dissatisfied		Fairly Dissatisfied		A Little Dissatisfied		A Little Satisfied		Fairly Satisfied	Very Satisfied

7. List each significant person in your life. Consider all the persons who provide personal support for you or who are important to you now. Use only their first names or initials. Write the relationship of each person next to his or her initials (see example). Next, circle how satisfied you are with the support you have from that person in dealing with your pain.

EXAMPLE: O. U. (Brother)
             C. H. (Husband)
             I. E. (Friend)

	Very Dissatisfied			**Moderately Dissatisfied**			**Moderately Satisfied**			**Very Satisfied**
_____	1	2	3	4	5	6	7	8	9	10
_____	1	2	3	4	5	6	7	8	9	10
_____	1	2	3	4	5	6	7	8	9	10
_____	1	2	3	4	5	6	7	8	9	10
_____	1	2	3	4	5	6	7	8	9	10
_____	1	2	3	4	5	6	7	8	9	10
_____	1	2	3	4	5	6	7	8	9	10
_____	1	2	3	4	5	6	7	8	9	10
_____	1	2	3	4	5	6	7	8	9	10
_____	1	2	3	4	5	6	7	8	9	10

Scoring: Add up your responses to questions 1-6, inverting the scores for questions 2 and 3 (e.g., 10 = 1, 9 = 2, 8 = 3, etc.). Add up the ratings on question 7 and divide by the number of persons. Add the average score from 7 to the total score from 1-6. Divide by 7 and this will be your final score.

The following scale can be used to measure your level of perceived support:

Greater than 9	=	excellent support
Between 8 and 9	=	adequate support
Between 6 and 8	=	moderate support
Less than 6	=	poor support

The most important points in this chapter that I want to remember are . . .

1. _____

_____

_____

_____

_____

_____

2. _____

_____

_____

_____

_____

_____

3. _____

_____

_____

_____

_____

_____

Chapter 21

HOW TO PREVENT RELAPSE

OVERVIEW

One of the frustrating aspects of dealing with your pain is that you have setbacks. This chapter explores ways that you can plan for future setbacks and prevent having a relapse.

INTRODUCTION

Like all people with chronic pain, you will have good and bad days. The important thing is to prevent a lapse - a slip or a step backward in which your progress is stalled for a short time - from becoming a relapse into chronic disability. The goals in preventing a relapse are (a) to maintain a steady level of exercise, relaxation, and appropriate use of medication; and (b) to anticipate and deal with situations that can cause setbacks before they bring on a relapse.

TWO SCENARIOS

SCENARIO #1

Joe is having a bad day. He decides not to exercise. He becomes depressed and stays in bed the next day. After 2 days of inactivity, he feels stiff and notices an increase in the intensity of his pain; therefore, he again decides that it would be best to remain inactive. Again he feels so depressed and discouraged that he does not leave the house. He takes some of the pain medication that he has been saving for particularly bad days. After using up his supply of medication, he calls his doctor to get another prescription. Soon he is having the same problems that he has had in the past: increased pain, reliance on medication, physical weakness, and depression.

SCENARIO #2

Sally is having a bad day. She decides to do some of her exercises but also to allow herself longer periods of rest. Although feeling discouraged and admitting to herself that she is having a bad day, she recognizes that better days are ahead. She sets goals for getting back to her full program gradually over the next 3 days. She keeps her mind occupied and uses some relaxation techniques without overly relying on medication. Over the next 3 days, she gradually feels better about herself as she returns to her regular exercise program. What may have been the beginning of a relapse turns out to be a simple lapse.

KEY QUESTIONS

Here are some questions that may help you focus on responding to pain in a manner that prevents you from falling back into inactivity, depression, and/or overreliance on medication. Take time to answer each of these questions:

1. How do I view a lapse?
2. Do I consider a bad day evidence of failure, signaling that I will now return to my lowest point?
3. Am I especially hard on myself when my pain is worse? (Do I blame myself when I cannot do everything the way I used to or when I need more rest than usual?)
4. How good am I at sticking with a resolution to change a particular behavior?
5. Where do I go to get help when I'm having a bad day?

Complete the Relapse Prevention Worksheet on page 191. Refer to your answers on those occasions when you experience a flare-up of your pain.

STEPS IN PREVENTING
A RELAPSE

1. Make gradual progress toward resuming your full treatment program.
2. Continue to develop the skills you have learned (exercise, relaxation, monitoring of pain and medication).

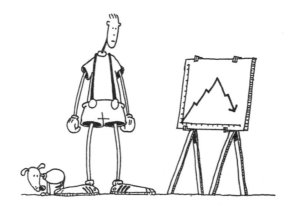

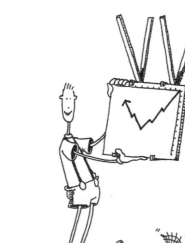

3. Replace negative habits (such as overreliance on medication) with positive ones (such as exercise and distraction).
4. Use your new skills for all stressors and problems (assertiveness, relaxation).
5. Develop an active and realistic plan to carry out all your new skills on a regular basis.
6. Recognize that you will have setbacks. Be ready to deal with them and get back on track.
7. Deal with setbacks as learning opportunities, not failures.
8. Maintain contact with health professionals and with other people with chronic pain who are also working to maintain their gains.

<u>Relapse Prevention Worksheet</u>

1. What are my initial signals of a lapse? When is a lapse most likely to happen?

   _____

   _____

   _____

   _____

2. What did I do in the past that got me into further difficulty (closer to relapse)?

   _____

   _____

   _____

   _____

3. What will I do when I have a lapse the next time?

   _____

   _____

   _____

   _____

4. What will I do if #3 does not work?

   _____

   _____

   _____

   _____

The most important points in this chapter that I want to remember are . . .

1. _____

   _____

   _____

   _____

   _____

2. _____

   _____

   _____

   _____

   _____

3. _____

   _____

   _____

   _____

   _____

Chapter 22

WHAT TO DO TO
MAINTAIN THE GAINS

OVERVIEW

This is a quick review of what you have learned and what you can do to keep improving your condition.

INTRODUCTION

The goals outlined in this book are to reduce your pain intensity, increase your physical capacity, improve your mood, and give you more control of your situation. By now you have learned a great deal about how to manage your pain physically and emotionally, despite some ups and downs. To carry the benefits of this training with you and to live a more satisfying life with less pain, you will need to practice the strategies you have learned every day. Review the following list periodically:

1. *Continue With Your Exercise Program.* Exercise a little every day. Try to stick with the exercises suggested by your physical therapist and exercise physiologist.
2. *Keep Records.* Create your own charts to graph your progress in your exercise program. In addition, use the forms in your booklet to monitor your thoughts, moods, and pain-intensity ratings.

3. *Watch Your Body Cues.* Be aware of excess muscle tension and other signs of stress and tension.

4. *Use Relaxation.* Practice your relaxation techniques, using a relaxation tape or following the cue-controlled relaxation strategies.

5. *Stick to a Schedule.* Set aside specific times every day to practice relaxation and to exercise.

6. *Find Time for Yourself.* Remember that you need time just to enjoy yourself. Guard your personal time. Resist jumping back into your old routine.

7. *Pace Yourself.* Take breaks during long tasks. Have a fallback plan for days that are particularly difficult. Remember to set some limits on your activities.

8. *Watch Your Diet.* Eat wisely. Use a sensible diet if you are trying to lose weight.

9. *Get Involved in Activities.* Stay as active as possible and keep your mind stimulated.

10. *Contact Other People for Help.* Ask for support when you need it by contacting friends and family members or other persons with chronic pain.

11. *Express Your Emotions.* Talk to others about your feelings. Find ways to vent your emotions in constructive ways.

12. *Seek Professional Help.* On those occasions when you are overwhelmed and need guidance consult with a professional for direction and feedback.

Complete the Follow-Up Plan of Care form on page 213. Discuss with your case manager, therapist, and family members your plans for maintaining the gains you have made.

The most important points in this chapter that I want to remember are

1. _____

   _____

   _____

   _____

   _____

   _____

2. _____

   _____

   _____

   _____

   _____

   _____

3. _____

   _____

   _____

   _____

   _____

   _____

APPENDICES

APPENDIX A

Daily Pain Rating Scale

Directions: The top half of each block is for your estimated degree of pain in the morning and should be completed by lunchtime. The bottom half of each block is for your estimated degree of pain in the afternoon and evening and should be completed before bedtime.

EXAMPLE:

	Scale:	0	=	No Pain
		1-2	=	Mild
Date: ²/₁₀		3-4	=	Moderate
Day 5		5-6	=	Intense, Severe
A.M. [2]		7-8	=	Very Intense, Horrible
P.M. [5]		9-10	=	Excruciating, Unbearable

Date: _____

	Day 1	Day 2	Day 3	Day 4	Day 5	Day 6	Day 7
A.M.							
P.M.							

Date: _____

	Day 8	Day 9	Day 10	Day 11	Day 12	Day 13	Day 14
A.M.							
P.M.							

Date: _____

	Day 15	Day 16	Day 17	Day 18	Day 19	Day 20	Day 21
A.M.							
P.M.							

Date: _____

	Day 22	Day 23	Day 24	Day 25	Day 26	Day 27	Day 28
A.M.							
P.M.							

APPENDIX B

Daily Activity Record

Name:_____Date:_____

Day of the Week: _____

Directions: This record is useful for monitoring the pattern of your activity, medication use, and pain intensity throughout the day. Enter the number of minutes you spend sitting, standing/walking, or reclining each hour. Record every time you take pain-related medication and monitor your hourly pain intensity.

Time	Sitting	Standing and Walking	Reclining (Put "S" if Sleeping)	Medication (Name and Quantity)	Pain (0-10) (None to Unbearable)
A.M.					
06-07					
07-08					
08-09					
09-10					
10-11					
11-12					
P.M.					
12-01					
01-02					
02-03					
03-04					
04-05					
05-06					
06-07					
07-08					

Time	Sitting	Standing and Walking	Reclining (Put "S" if Sleeping)	Medication (Name and Quantity)	Pain (0-10) (None to Unbearable)
P.M. *(Continued)*					
08-09					
09-10					
10-11					
11-12					
A.M.					
12-01					
01-02					
02-03					
03-04					
04-05					
05-06					

APPENDIX C

Weekly Activity Record

Directions: Please fill out this sheet for the next 7 days. The hours should add up to 24 each day.

Date	Hours spent walking or standing	Hours spent sitting	Hours spent reclining (both feet off the floor)
Monday			
Tuesday			
Wednesday			
Thursday			
Friday			
Saturday			
Sunday			

APPENDIX D

Exercise Record

Name: _____

Start Date: _____ Record #: _____

Directions: This form should be used to monitor your exercise. Please circle whether you stretched before and after each exercise session. Include the date and type of exercise and check the combined time you spent exercising.

Day	1	2	3	4	5	6	7	8	9	10
Warm-Up Stretching	Y	Y	Y	Y	Y	Y	Y	Y	Y	Y
Cool-Down Stretching	Y	Y	Y	Y	Y	Y	Y	Y	Y	Y

```
           20  .   .   .   .   .   .   .   .   .   .
Minutes
of Cardio- 15  .   .   .   .   .   .   .   .   .   .
vascular
Activity   10  .   .   .   .   .   .   .   .   .   .

            5  .   .   .   .   .   .   .   .   .   .

            0  .   .   .   .   .   .   .   .   .   .

Date:          __  __  __  __  __  __  __  __  __  __
```

Activity:

APPENDIX E

Medication Record

Name: _____ Date: _____

Directions: Please fill out this sheet for the next 7 days. List all the drugs you take each day, the milligrams (mg), and the number of pills or capsules you take per day. List any "over-the-counter" drugs you take, such as aspirin, Bufferin, Tylenol, and so forth.

Date	Name of Drug	Number of Milligrams (mg)	Number of Pills or Capsules Taken Each Day
Monday			
Tuesday			
Wednesday			

Date	Name of Drug	Number of Milligrams (mg)	Number of Pills or Capsules Taken Each Day
Thursday			
Friday			
Saturday			
Sunday			

APPENDIX F

Daily Food Diary

Name: _____   Date: _____

Directions: Please record everything that you eat throughout the day. Enter the time that you eat it, your level of hunger, a brief description of the food and amount, whether you ate it as part of a meal, and your level of pain.

	Time	Hunger* 1-5	Food Description	Amount	Meal (Y/N)	Pain 0-10
1.						
2.						
3.						
4.						
5.						
6.						

*1 = not hungry; 5 = extremely hungry

Time	Hunger* 1-5	Food Description	Amount	Meal (Y/N)	Pain 0-10
7.					
8.					
9.					
10.					
11.					
12.					
13.					
14.					
15.					

*1 = not hungry; 5 = extremely hungry

APPENDIX G

<u>Follow-Up Plan of Care</u>

For: _____

Finish Date: _____

I realize that I have made progress in this program because of what I have done. In order to keep what I have gained in this program and to go forward, I must make a commitment to keep doing all the things that have helped me improve. I am therefore making a commitment to continue with the following activities:

Exercise: _____
_____
_____
_____

Relaxation: _____
_____
_____
_____

Medications: _____
_____
_____
_____

Other: _____
_____
_____
_____

In addition, I will attend the follow-up sessions.

_____   _____
Patient   Case Manager

APPENDIX H

Americans With
Disabilities Act Outline

The following are highlights of the Americans With Disabilities Act (ADA), which all potential employers are legally required to follow.

RECRUITING AND SCREENING EMPLOYEES

*   Recruitment materials welcome applicants with disabilities.
*   Open hiring and promotion policies exist.
*   Vendor and subcontractor nondiscrimination requirements are posted.
*   Interviewing rooms are accessible to persons with disabilities.
*   All tests and selection criteria are related to a specific job and reflect essential skills and performance requirements for the job.
*   Applicants can get information about accessible testing policy.
*   Testing procedures can accommodate workers with disabilities.
*   Applications do not ask about disability.
*   Interviewers do not question nature or extent of disability; they focus strictly on job-related skills and abilities.

HIRING DECISIONS

*   Safety criteria relate strictly to mental or physical abilities that are essential to safe performance or essential job tasks.
*   Preemployment medical examinations are not required until after a conditional offer of employment has been made.
*   Medical examinations focus only on the specific mental and physical qualities that are necessary to perform the essential functions of a particular job.

ON THE JOB

*   Information about a worker's disability is kept confidential and shared with supervisors and safety personnel only on a need-to-know basis.
*   The employer has a reasonable accommodation policy that provides changes needed so that employees with known disabilities have an opportunity to perform the essential functions of their jobs effectively.

- Each employee's work site is arranged so that the employee can effectively perform the essential functions of his or her job.
- Employees and supervisors are informed about the reasonable accommodation process.
- The reasonable accommodation process operates on a case-by-case basis in a cooperative problem-solving manner with input from the individual employee.
- Facilities used by all employees are readily accessible to and usable by employees with disabilities, unless it is an undue hardship to do this.
- Job restructuring is an available, reasonable accommodation if necessary in a particular situation.
- Modified work schedules are available as a reasonable accommodation, if needed.
- Transfer or reassignment options are provided as reasonable accommodations, if necessary.
- Adaptive equipment is available as needed.
- Marginal job requirements are waivable in order to accommodate a worker's disability.
- The services of readers or interpreters are available for workers who require them.
- Benefits like insurance, sick leave, and leave of absence are as equally available to employees with disabilities as to their co-workers.

EMPLOYMENT DECISIONS

- Employees with disabilities have opportunities for promotion and advancement.
- Adverse employment actions are reviewed before implementation to ensure that there are legitimate business reasons for the action and that workers with a disability are not being unfairly penalized.
- A no-retaliation policy is known and followed for employees who grieve reasonable accommodation issues or other civil rights matters.
- A worker with a spouse or a family member who has a disability is not disadvantaged in employment decisions.

SUBJECT INDEX

A

Activity
    Activity List, 59-60
    Daily Activity Record, 203-204
    Weekly Activity Record, 205
Americans With Disabilities Act, 129-130, 215-216
Assertiveness Training, 93
    Improving Communication, 96-97
    Scenarios, 94-96
    Styles, Aggressive, 93
    Styles, Assertive, 94
    Styles, Passive, 94

B

Biofeedback, 14-15, 89
    Electrodermal Activity (EDA), 15
    Electromyographic Biofeedback (EMG), 14
    Peripheral Temperature (TEMP), 14-15
Body Mechanics, 37

C

Catastrophizing, 102, 151
Clothing and Posture, 39
    Clothing and Posture Worksheet, 57-58

G

H

I